Social-Emotional Assessment/Evaluation Measure (SEAM™)

Research Edition

Social-Emotional Assessment/Evaluation Measure (SEAM™)

Research Edition

by

Jane Squires, Ph.D.

Diane Bricker, Ph.D.

Misti Waddell, M.S.

Kristin Funk, M.A., LCSW

Jantina Clifford, Ph.D.

and

Robert Hoselton, B.S.

University of Oregon, Eugene

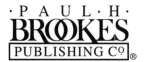

·P·A·U·L·H·
BROOKES
PUBLISHING C⁰ ®

Baltimore • London • Sydney

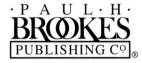

Paul H. Brookes Publishing Co.
Post Office Box 10624
Baltimore, Maryland 21285-0624

www.brookespublishing.com

Typeset by Cenveo, Inc., Stamford, Connecticut.
Manufactured in the United States of America by
Versa Press, East Peoria Illinois.

All of the case studies in this book are composites of the authors' actual experiences. In all instances, names and identifying details have been altered to protect confidentiality.

Social-Emotional Assessment/Evaluation Measure (SEAM™), Research Edition, can be purchased in print format (ISBN-13:978-1-59857-280-3) or can be purchased in PDF format (ISBN-13: 978-1-59857-718-1). To order, contact Brookes Publishing Co., 1-800-638-3775; www.brookespublishing.com.

Selected photographs in the forms that appear in *Social-Emotional Assessment/Evaluation Measure (SEAM™),
Research Edition,* by Jane Squires, Diane Bricker, Misti Waddell, Kristin Funk, Jantina Clifford, and Robert Hoselton are
© istockphoto/anatols, © istockphoto/lostinbids, © Veer/Fancy Photography, © istockphoto/Nick_Thompson,
© Fotosearch/Dex Images, © Blend Images/Ariel Skelley, © Veer/ampyang, © istockphoto/asiseeit, © Veer/Fancy
Photography, © istockphoto/AngiePhotos, and © istockphoto/theboone.

Library of Congress Cataloging-in-Publication Data
The Library of Congress has cataloged the print edition as follows:
Squires, Jane.
  Social-emotional assessment/evaluation measure (SEAM™), / by Jane Squires, Ph.D., Diane Bricker, Ph.D.,
  Misti Waddell, M.S., Kristin Funk, M.A., LCSW, Jantina Clifford, Ph.D., and Robert Hoselton, B.S—Research edition.
      pages   cm
  Includes bibliographical references and index.
  ISBN 978-1-59857-280-3 (pbk.) — ISBN 1-59857-280-6 (pbk.)
  1. Child development—Testing.   2. Psychological tests for children.   3. Child development deviations—Diagnosis.
  I. Bricker, Diane.   II. Waddell, Misti.   III. Funk, Kristen.   IV. Clifford, Jantina.   V. Hoselton, Robert.   VI. Title.
  RJ51.D48S65 2014
  618.92'85882—dc23   2013027814

British Library Cataloguing in Publication data are available from the British Library.

2018   2017   2016   2015   2014

10   9   8   7   6   5   4   3   2   1

Contents

About the SEAM™ CD-ROM

This book contains a CD-ROM with printable versions of the *Social-Emotional Assessment/Evaluation Measure (SEAM™), Research Edition*, forms. The CD-ROM includes SEAM™, SEAM™ with Ages, SEAM™ Family Profile, and SEAM™ Summary Forms (as well as additional generic cover sheets) in both English and Spanish.

Purchasers may print or photocopy the forms from a computer located within their own facilities at a single physical site in the course of their service provision. Refer to the End User License Agreement (EULA) on the CD-ROM for details.

All of the materials in the CD-ROM for this book (ISBN-13: 978-1-59857-280-3) are provided in PDF format. You may save these PDFs to your computer and/or post them on an internal local area network (LAN) for employees to print as needed, in accordance with the terms of the EULA that you accepted when you accessed the CD-ROM.

Selected photographs in the forms that appear in *Social-Emotional Assessment/Evaluation Measure (SEAM™), Research Edition,* by Jane Squires, Diane Bricker, Misti Waddell, Kristin Funk, Jantina Clifford, and Robert Hoselton are © istockphoto/anatols, © istockphoto/lostinbids, © Veer/Fancy Photography, © istockphoto/Nick_Thompson, © Fotosearch/Dex Images, © Blend Images/Ariel Skelley, © Veer/ampyang, © istockphoto/asiseeit, © Veer/Fancy Photography, © istockphoto/AngiePhotos, and © istockphoto/theboone.

Contents of the SEAM™ CD-ROM

Generic Cover Sheets
SEAM™ generic cover sheet
SEAM™ Spanish generic cover sheet
SEAM™ Family Profile generic cover sheet
SEAM™ Formulario para familias generic cover sheet

End User License Agreement

About the Authors

Jane Squires, Ph.D., Professor, Early Intervention Program, Center on Human Development, College of Education, 5253 University of Oregon, Eugene, Oregon 97403

Dr. Squires is Director of the Early Intervention Program at the University of Oregon and Director of the University Center for Excellence in Developmental Disabilities and the Center on Human Development. Dr. Squires oversees research and outreach projects in the areas of developmental screening, implementation of screening systems, early identification of developmental delays, and the involvement of parents in monitoring their young children's development. She is coauthor of the *Ages & Stages Questionnaires®: A Parent-Completed Child Monitoring System, Third Edition* (with D. Bricker; Paul H. Brookes Publishing Co., 2009), and *Ages & Stages Questionnaires®: Social-Emotional* (with D. Bricker & E. Twombly; Paul H. Brookes Publishing Co., 2002) and has authored or coauthored more than 90 books, chapters, assessments, videotapes, and articles on developmental screening and assessment, personnel preparation, and early childhood disabilities.

Diane Bricker, Ph.D., Professor Emerita, Early Intervention Program, Center on Human Development, College of Education, 5253 University of Oregon, Eugene, Oregon 97403

Dr. Bricker received her bachelor's degree from The Ohio State University, her master's degree in special education at the University of Oregon, and her doctoral degree in special education from Vanderbilt University, Peabody College. Her initial work focused on improving the language skills of children with severe disabilities in institutions. That work led to the development of one of the first community-based integrated early intervention programs in the early 1970s. Since then, her work has continued in the area of early intervention, including her work on the *Ages & Stages Questionnaires®: A Parent-Completed Child Monitoring System, Third Edition* (with J. Squires; Paul H. Brookes Publishing Co., 2009); *Ages & Stages Questionnaires®: Social-Emotional* (with J. Squires & E. Twombly; Paul H. Brookes Publishing Co., 2002); *Assessment, Evaluation, and Programming System for Infants and Children (AEPS®), Second Edition* (Bricker et al.; Paul H. Brookes Publishing Co., 2002); and *An Activity-Based Approach to Early Intervention, Third Edition* (with K. Pretti-Frontzcak; Paul H. Brookes Publishing Co., 2004). Dr. Bricker has directed a number of national demonstration projects and research examining the efficacy of early intervention; the development of a linked assessment, goal development, intervention, and evaluation system; and the study of a comprehensive, parent-completed screening measure. Dr. Bricker has also directed a graduate training program focused on preparing early interventionists. More than 300 students have received their master's or doctoral degrees from this program and have gone on to practice in the field. Dr. Bricker served for 8 years as Associate Dean for Academic Programs in the College of Education at the University of Oregon.

Misti Waddell, M.S., Senior Research Assistant and Project Coordinator, Early Intervention Program, Center on Human Development, College of Education, 5253 University of Oregon, Eugene, Oregon 97403

In addition to coordinating research projects, Ms. Waddell has contributed to the development and research of the *Assessment, Evaluation, and Programming System for Infants and Children (AEPS®), Second Edition* (Bricker et al.; Paul H. Brookes Publishing Co., 2002), a curriculum-based assessment for young children. Her research projects include Project SEAM: Preventing Behavior Disorders and Improving Social Emotional Competence in Infants and Toddlers with Disabilities and Infant Mental Health: Improving Mental Health in Infants and Toddlers with Disabilities. Ms. Waddell provides field supervision for early intervention graduate students and has conducted training with early childhood teachers and parents in developmental and social-emotional screening, assessment, and intervention, including *AEPS*; *Ages & Stages Questionnaires®: A Parent-Completed Child Monitoring System, Third Edition* (Squires & Bricker; Paul H. Brookes Publishing Co., 2009); and *Ages & Stages Questionnaires®: Social-Emotional* (Squires, Bricker, & Twombly; Paul H. Brookes Publishing Co., 2002).

Kristin Funk, M.A., LCSW, Senior Research Assistant and Project Coordinator, Early Intervention Program, Center on Human Development, College of Education, 5253 University of Oregon, Eugene, Oregon 97403

Ms. Funk is a licensed clinical social worker who has worked on and coordinated several community-based systems-change grants and research projects, including Project SEAM: Preventing Behavior Disorders and Improving Social Emotional Competence in Infants and Toddlers with Disabilities, a 5-year research project to conduct psychometric studies for validation of the Social-Emotional Assessment/Evaluation Measure (SEAM™). She has conducted extensive training with early childhood teachers and parents in implementing social-emotional curricula and developmental and social-emotional screening, assessment, and intervention, including the *Assessment, Evaluation, and Programming System for Infants and Children (AEPS®), Second Edition* (Bricker et al., Paul H. Brookes Publishing Co., 2002); *Ages & Stages Questionnaires®: A Parent-Completed Child Monitoring System, Third Edition* (Squires & Bricker; Paul H. Brookes Publishing Co., 2009); and *Ages & Stages Questionnaires®: Social-Emotional* (Squires, Bricker, & Twombly; Paul H. Brookes Publishing Co., 2002).

Jantina Clifford, Ph.D., Assistant Professor, Early Intervention Program, Center on Human Development, College of Education, 5253 University of Oregon, Eugene, Oregon 97403

Dr. Clifford is Assistant Professor at the University of Oregon Early Intervention Program, where she teaches graduate courses in early intervention and early childhood special education. In addition to teaching at the university level, Dr. Clifford provides training internationally on the *Ages & Stages Questionnaires®: A Parent-Completed Child Monitoring System, Third Edition* (Squires & Bricker; Paul H. Brookes Publishing Co., 2009), and the *Ages & Stages Questionnaires®: Social-Emotional* (Squires, Bricker, & Twombly; Paul H. Brookes Publishing Co., 2002). Her professional interests include personnel preparation and the development and evaluation of early childhood assessment measures. Prior to the pursuit of her doctoral degree, Dr. Clifford served as an early childhood educator for 8 years.

Robert Hoselton, B.S., Research Assistant, Early Intervention Program, Center on Human Development, 5253 University of Oregon, Eugene, Oregon 97403

Mr. Hoselton received a B.S. degree in computer science from the University of Oregon in 2004. He has been involved with several research studies on the *Ages & Stages Questionnaires® (ASQ): A Parent-Completed Child Monitoring System, Third Edition* (with J. Squires; Paul H. Brookes Publishing Co., 2009) and the Social-Emotional Assessment/Evaluation Measure (SEAM™). His most important contributions include data collection and analysis for technical reports. Mr. Hoselton designed and developed web applications used for national ASQ and SEAM data collection.

Acknowledgments

The quality and usefulness of assessment and curricular materials for young children such as the Social-Emotional Assessment/Evaluation Measure (SEAM™) is dependent on the conceptual organization, hard work, and tenacity of their developers and, more important, on the willingness of others to contribute time, ideas, information, and data. We wish to thank and acknowledge the contributors whose input has done much to improve the SEAM. First, we wish to thank and acknowledge the many family members who participated in data collection efforts designed to improve the SEAM. These family members and their children provided an array of feedback and information that was incorporated into SEAM revisions. Second, we wish to thank and acknowledge the host of practitioners who cheered us on and offered constructive feedback that has done much to improve the SEAM. Third, we wish to thank and acknowledge a group of special colleagues who were essential to the research efforts that examined the validity, reliability, and utility of the SEAM. These colleagues include Marisa Macy and her steadfast data collection efforts in Pennsylvania; Kimberly Murphy, who tirelessly recruited online data participants; and Erin Barton, who assisted us in initial data collection and ongoing training efforts. Fourth, we wish to thank and acknowledge the enormous contribution made by University of Oregon Early Intervention doctoral students (now Ph.D.s!) Ching I-Chen, Lois Pribble, Maria Pomes, Aoife Magee, Mona Ivey-Soto, and Kathy Moxley. As all university-based researchers know, doctoral students provide critically important and affordable assistance in data collection, analysis, and translation activities. Finally, we wish to thank and acknowledge Annette Tognazzini for her patience, perseverance, and document-creation skills.

To the many individuals who were critical to the development,
testing, and refinement of the SEAM™. First, we thank
the hundreds of families who participated in our research and
used the SEAM with their infants, toddlers, and preschool children
to give us vital feedback and suggestions for improvement.
The data provided by these caregivers and hundreds of babies and children
helped to support the validity of the SEAM and its components. Second, we thank
a wide array of practitioners who were enthusiastic about the SEAM
from its inception and were invaluable to the development of procedures,
refinement of items, and revisions. Their dedication, energy, and
collaborative efforts throughout the development process made it possible.

1

Introduction to the SEAM™

The Social-Emotional Assessment/Evaluation Measure (SEAM™) is a functional tool for assessing and monitoring social-emotional and behavioral development in infants, toddlers, and preschoolers at risk for social-emotional delays or problems. The SEAM was developed to assist in the early identification of social-emotional difficulties and behavior disorders and to prevent problems by building positive partnerships with families and optimizing positive parent–child interactions in the first years of life. It is designed for use by a variety of professionals, including those without a background or training in mental health and/or behavioral interventions. The SEAM system was designed to be administered in a child's home, child care center, intervention program, and other community settings in order to yield in-depth information on children's social-emotional skills and deficits as well as their caregivers' strengths and areas of need. Such information can be used by child care workers, teachers, and early intervention or early childhood special education personnel to develop high-quality and developmentally appropriate social-emotional goals and objectives for children and their families. The United States has seen increasing variations in children's family constellations and who takes care of children. Consequently, we have chosen to use the word *caregiver* throughout the guide to include parents, guardians, child care workers, or other familiar people who provide care and attention to the infant or child on a regular basis.

SEAM results can contribute to developing and selecting intervention goals and objectives once an assessment of a child's social-emotional competence is completed. Selected goals and objectives can then guide intervention efforts. The SEAM can be used as part of a linked activity-based social-emotional assessment system described by Squires and Bricker (2007).

The SEAM can be used to track children's progress toward acquiring selected social-emotional goals once intervention activities are undertaken. Finally, the SEAM can be used in tandem with screening instruments such as the Ages & Stages Questionnaires®: Social-Emotional (ASQ:SE; Squires, Bricker, & Twombly, 2002) and the Infant Toddler Social Emotional Assessment (ITSEA; Carter & Briggs-Gowan, 2006) or other available early detection measures.

WHAT ARE THE COMPONENTS OF THE SEAM™ SYSTEM?

The SEAM system is designed to evaluate young children's social-emotional and behavioral development and to offer linked intervention ideas and content for prevention and habilitation activities

Table 1.1.   The Social-Emotional Assessment/Evaluation Measure (SEAM™) system

Title	Developmental intervals	Focus	Who completes it?
SEAM	Infant (2–18 months) Toddler (18–36 months) Preschool (36–66 months)	Child	Caregivers
SEAM with Ages	Infant (2–18 months) Toddler (18–36 months) Preschool (36–66 months)	Child	Used by child care practitioners to guide caregiver completion of the SEAM
SEAM Family Profile	Infant (2–18 months) Toddler (18–36 months) Preschool (36–66 months)	Caregiver	Caregivers

All forms are available in Spanish.

particularly focused on developing the social-emotional competence of young children. The SEAM system is composed of three components—SEAM, SEAM with Ages, and SEAM Family Profile (see Table 1.1). The SEAM has three developmental intervals—Infant, Toddler, and Preschool. The SEAM with Ages parallels the content of the SEAM and also includes chronological age ranges for item examples. The SEAM Family Profile also has three developmental intervals and is designed to assess caregiver strengths, concerns, and needs for additional support and resources. Each component is described in detail in this guide. All components are included on the accompanying CD-ROM (for print users) or as part of the PDF e-book (for digital users) in both English and Spanish.

SEAM™ Spanish Translation

All SEAM forms have been translated into Spanish to better serve Spanish-speaking families and practitioners who work with Spanish-speaking children. The translation team consisted of two individuals, one native Spanish speaker from Mexico and one native English speaker. Both have lived in Mexico, have extensive experience teaching Spanish, and have translated a wide variety of materials from Spanish to English and vice versa. Once the translation was complete, the Spanish version of the SEAM forms was reviewed by another Spanish-speaking early childhood professional and parent from Chile. The original translators then conducted a final review.

The translated SEAM forms closely follow the original English version using standard Spanish to the extent possible. A few cultural representations have been altered to better correspond to Latino culture. For example, Item 1.5 in the Preschool Interval of the SEAM (Child shares and takes turns with other children) includes examples of games in which children might take turns (e.g., Red Rover). Names of games common in Latino culture are included in the Spanish translation of this item (e.g., *Martín pescador*). When foods are used in examples, the Spanish translation includes foods common in Spanish-speaking families. The translators chose to use the word or structure most prevalent in Mexican Spanish in cases in which multiple translations could convey the meaning of an item. The language usage on the SEAM forms will therefore be familiar to Mexican Spanish speakers.

Spanish forms were completed during the research study described in Chapter 7, Technical Report. Spanish forms were used by a small number ($n = 29$) of Spanish-speaking practitioners and caregivers in Georgia, Pennsylvania, and Oregon. This number was not large enough to conduct a separate study to determine whether English and Spanish forms functioned in a similar manner. Spanish-speaking practitioners and caregivers were included in utility studies, however, and focus group data includes feedback from users of the Spanish forms. If you have any feedback or questions about the Spanish translation of SEAM, please contact the developers at jsquires@uoregon.edu.

SEAM™ FEEDBACK

This manual is a research edition; work on the tool is ongoing. Please contact the developers at jsquires@uoregon.edu to provide feedback on the SEAM.

2

SEAM™

The SEAM includes three intervals: *Infant*, with a developmental range of 2–18 months; *Toddler*, with a developmental range of 18–36 months; and *Preschool*, with a developmental range of 36–66 months. The Infant, Toddler, and Preschool Intervals refer to children's developmental competency rather than their chronological age. This distinction is particularly important for children with disabilities who may have a significant discrepancy between their chronological age and their developmental skills. It is important to begin at the child's developmental level when undertaking intervention efforts.

The standard cover sheet for each SEAM interval indicates the name of the interval (i.e., Infant, Toddler, Preschool) and the developmental range for each interval (see Figure 2.1 for an example of the standard cover sheet for the Infant Interval). An alternate cover sheet without the interval and developmental range is also available (see Figure 2.2). For example, a program that serves children with severe developmental delays may decide to use the alternate cover sheet when giving it to caregivers to complete because a toddler with significant developmental delays may demonstrate social-emotional skills and behaviors that are addressed in the Infant Interval, rather than the Toddler Interval, of the SEAM. Generic cover sheets are also available for users to photocopy and use.

Each SEAM interval is composed of 10 benchmarks with corresponding behavioral items to be assessed and scored. Benchmarks and corresponding items represent social-emotional and behavioral competence skills that children need in order to meet their own needs, develop a sense of self, successfully participate in a range of home and community activities, regulate their emotions, and engage in positive interactions with peers, siblings, parents, and other adults (Squires & Bricker, 2007). Understanding appropriate social-emotional development in young children and targeting appropriate goals are complex undertakings. The complexity stems from the need to view social-emotional responses of children through at least three important lenses. First, the appropriateness of responses or reactions depends on the developmental age or stage of the child. Appropriateness is often tied to age expectations; that is, expectations for infants generally are far different from those of preschool-age children. Second, the context or setting helps set the parameter of appropriateness. Acceptable behavior on the playground is often different from acceptable behavior in a restaurant. Third, family and community values and expectations affect what others find appropriate. Some families and cultures find noisy, active children acceptable, whereas others do not. Consequently, defining and targeting appropriate social-emotional behavior for children is often more challenging than doing so for other areas of

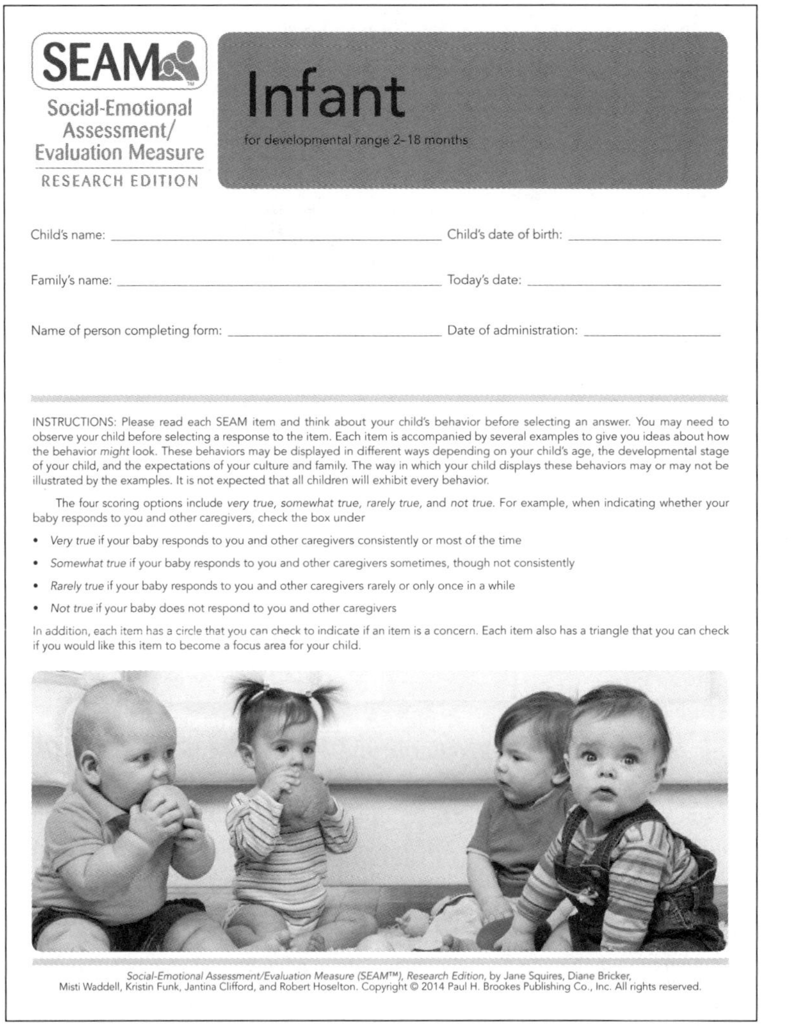

SEAM™

Social-Emotional Assessment/ Evaluation Measure

RESEARCH EDITION

Infant

for developmental range 2–18 months

Child's name: ______________________ Child's date of birth: ______________

Family's name: ______________________ Today's date: ______________

Name of person completing form: ______________ Date of administration: ______________

INSTRUCTIONS: Please read each SEAM item and think about your child's behavior before selecting an answer. You may need to observe your child before selecting a response to the item. Each item is accompanied by several examples to give you ideas about how the behavior *might* look. These behaviors may be displayed in different ways depending on your child's age, the developmental stage of your child, and the expectations of your culture and family. The way in which your child displays these behaviors may or may not be illustrated by the examples. It is not expected that all children will exhibit every behavior.

The four scoring options include *very true, somewhat true, rarely true,* and *not true.* For example, when indicating whether your baby responds to you and other caregivers, check the box under

- *Very true* if your baby responds to you and other caregivers consistently or most of the time
- *Somewhat true* if your baby responds to you and other caregivers sometimes, though not consistently
- *Rarely true* if your baby responds to you and other caregivers rarely or only once in a while
- *Not true* if your baby does not respond to you and other caregivers

In addition, each item has a circle that you can check to indicate if an item is a concern. Each item also has a triangle that you can check if you would like this item to become a focus area for your child.

Figure 2.1. Sample of a standard cover sheet for the Social-Emotional Assessment/Evaluation Measure (SEAM™).

development. SEAM content attempts to recognize this reality, but the user should continually be aware of the need to evaluate the appropriateness of social-emotional responses for individual children and their families.

The number of items varies across benchmarks and intervals. For example, Benchmark 2.0 on the Infant Interval of the SEAM (Baby expresses a range of emotions) has three corresponding items, whereas Benchmark 10.0 on the Preschool Interval of the SEAM (Preschool-age child shows a range of adaptive skills) has seven corresponding items. Table 2.1 includes a list of all Infant Interval benchmarks and associated items. A complete list of SEAM benchmarks and items can be found in Appendix A.

Each item is accompanied by several examples in order to assist caregivers in completing the SEAM and to give families ideas about how their child might demonstrate the behavior. Item 2.1 (Baby smiles at you) includes the following examples of how a baby might exhibit this behavior:

- Smiles when you smile at him
- Smiles when you talk to him

Figure 2.3 shows a sample benchmark from the Toddler Interval, with corresponding items and examples. Each child benchmark on the SEAM is designated with *C* and the associated benchmark

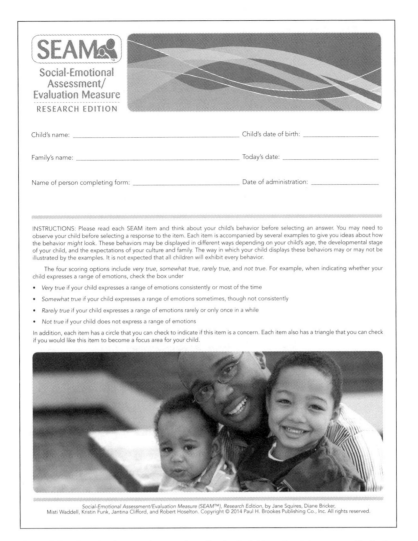

Figure 2.2. Sample of a generic cover sheet for the Social-Emotional Assessment/Evaluation Measure (SEAM™).

number (e.g., C-1.0). Corresponding items are designated with the benchmark number followed by item number and separated by a period (e.g., 1.1, 1.2, 1.3).

The SEAM does not include chronological age ranges for items or examples. Chronological ages were intentionally omitted from the SEAM to assist caregivers to focus on their child's actual behavior and developmental skills without being unduly influenced by suggested ages. We believe that caregivers of children with delayed development may benefit more from a focus on their child's individual strengths and emerging skills than from general age-based developmental expectations. The SEAM with Ages does contain age ranges for item examples to guide professionals in their work with families.

GUIDELINES FOR COMPLETING THE SEAM™

The SEAM is intended to include caregivers as partners in the assessment process to the greatest extent possible. It is important to remember, however, that the needs and values of caregivers may vary, affecting how each caregiver may choose to participate in the assessment process. Several methods are available for completing the SEAM, including independent completion (e.g., by caregivers), interview format, and joint completion (e.g., by caregiver and practitioner). Practitioners should tailor caregiver participation when possible to match the caregiver's individual needs and

Table 2.1. Benchmarks and items from the Infant Interval of the Social-Emotional Assessment/Evaluation Measure (SEAM™)

Benchmark	Item
C-1.0 Baby participates in healthy interactions	1.1 Baby shows interest in you and other familiar caregivers. 1.2 Baby lets you know if she needs help or comfort. 1.3 Baby responds to you and other family caregivers. 1.4 Baby initiates and responds to communications.
C-2.0 Baby expresses a range of emotions	2.1 Baby smiles at you. 2.2 Baby smiles at familiar people. 2.3 Baby smiles and laughs at sights and sounds.
C-3.0 Baby regulates own social-emotional responses with caregiver support	3.1 Baby calms down after exciting activity. 3.2 Baby responds to your soothing when upset. 3.3 Baby soothes self when distressed.
C-4.0 Baby begins to show empathy for others	4.1 Baby mimics your facial expression. 4.2 Baby looks at and notices you and other familiar caregivers. 4.3 Baby looks at and notices others' emotional responses. 4.4 Baby responds to another's distress, seeking comfort for self.
C-5.0 Baby attends to and engages with others	5.1 Baby looks at or toward sounds and visual events. 5.2 Baby makes eye contact with you and others. 5.3 Baby focuses on events shown by you and others. 5.4 Baby shares attention and events with you.
C-6.0 Baby explores hands and feet and surroundings	6.1 Baby explores hands and feet. 6.2 Baby explores toys and materials. 6.3 Baby explores surroundings. 6.4 Baby crawls or walks a short distance away from you.
C-7.0 Baby displays a positive self-image	7.1 Baby calls attention to self. 7.2 Baby laughs or smiles at own image or picture of self. 7.3 Baby recognizes own name.
C-8.0 Baby regulates activity level	8.1 Baby participates in simple routines and games with you. 8.2 Baby engages in motor activities for several minutes or longer. 8.3 Baby looks at books or pictures for several minutes or longer.
C-9.0 Baby cooperates with daily routines and requests	9.1 Baby opens mouth for food. 9.2 Baby follows simple routines with your help. 9.3 Baby cooperates with diaper and clothing changes.
C-10.0 Baby shows a range of adaptive skills	10.1 Baby eliminates (pees and poops) on regular schedule. 10.2 Baby eats and gains weight on schedule. 10.3 Baby sleeps with few problems. 10.4 Baby eats a variety of age-appropriate foods.

desires. They can provide caregivers with a copy of the SEAM to independently complete or recommend that caregivers jointly complete the tool with a practitioner, depending on the caregivers' language and literacy level. Practitioners can also administer the SEAM in the context of parent groups or classes, reviewing SEAM questions aloud as caregivers follow along and score items. An interview format is the method of completion preferred by many practitioners because it allows them to clarify items, explain examples, explore concerns, and assist caregivers in choosing appropriate response options. If caregiver completion of the SEAM is not possible, or if practitioners want to compare their experience of a child with that of a caregiver, then practitioners can also complete a separate SEAM.

As mentioned previously, it is important to be sensitive to each family's individual issues and needs. Special consideration should be given to introducing the SEAM to families when practitioners have serious concerns about a child and the family is not aware of those concerns. Practitioners are advised to use sensitivity when deciding whether to ask families to independently complete the SEAM. They may decide to complete the SEAM in an interview in cases in which they believe that the SEAM will reveal new information that might be emotionally difficult for a family to understand and accept. Practitioners can then be available to provide support and immediately respond to caregiver concerns.

	Very true	Somewhat true	Rarely true	Not true	Concern	Focus area
C-1.0 TODDLER PARTICIPATES IN HEALTHY INTERACTIONS						
1.1 Toddler lets you know if he needs help, attention, or comfort.	☐	☐	☐	☐	○	△

Some examples might be
  Asks for a drink of water by pointing or showing you
  Pulls on you or other adult or raises arms to be picked up
  Goes to you or other familiar adults when hurt
  Seeks attention from you and other familiar adults; babbles and "shows off" for you
  Asks for a drink of water using one- or two-word utterances
  Calls for you when he needs help (e.g., "Daddy help")

1.2 Toddler initiates and responds to affection.	☐	☐	☐	☐	○	△

Some examples might be
  Comes when you ask or gesture for her to follow
  Hugs you; smiles back at you
  Hugs and kisses people, pets, and stuffed animals
  Returns hugs, kisses, or other affectionate gestures
  Walks to you with arms out, wanting a hug

1.3 Toddler talks and plays with people whom he knows well.	☐	☐	☐	☐	○	△

Some examples might be
  Points to show you things
  Begins to include you or siblings in play, pretends to offer you or others food, tries to care for baby sibling or dolls
  Uses one or two words to communicate with peers (e.g., "Car go?")
  Talks to you about his activities (e.g., "I push car")

1.4 Toddler initiates and responds when you communicate with her.	☐	☐	☐	☐	○	△

Some examples might be
  Answers your questions with one word (e.g., "juice")
  Asks questions (e.g., "Where mama?"), says, "Mama come" when she wants you to play
  Asks many questions (e.g., "Why?" "What?" "How?")

Figure 2.3.   Benchmark 1.0 from the Toddler Interval of the Social-Emotional Assessment/Evaluation Measure (SEAM™).

Introducing the SEAM™ to Caregivers

It is ideal for a practitioner to have time to build a relationship with a caregiver and establish a base of mutual trust and understanding before beginning the assessment. It may take several visits or interactions before caregivers feel comfortable sharing concerns related to their child as well as their own issues and concerns. Cultural values, family demands, child-rearing practices, and personal characteristics may also affect how caregivers answer the assessment questions. Although not always possible, it is recommended that practitioners make several home visits or classroom contacts to build mutual trust before they ask caregivers to help complete the SEAM. If a practitioner does not have a chance to visit the caregiver beforehand, however, the SEAM could be used to help develop the relationship and to choose initial goals for intervention.

The first step of SEAM completion is to explain to caregivers the purpose of the assessment process. Following is an example of how a practitioner might introduce the SEAM to caregivers.

"The SEAM is a tool that helps us take a look at your child's social-emotional development. Items on the SEAM focus on skills children need in order to get along well with others, control their own emotions and behaviors, and develop a positive self-image. The SEAM can help us identify specific skills and behaviors we can work on with your child, and it can also help us find resources to support your child's social-emotional development. Positive social-emotional skills help children to be successful in all areas of their lives."

Scoring Guidelines for SEAM™

Practitioners should review possible item response options with caregivers after introducing the SEAM and before caregivers complete it. As shown in Figure 2.3, SEAM intervals include four possible response options. Caregivers can check the box under *very true* if their child exhibits the behavior consistently or most of the time; *somewhat true* if their child exhibits the behavior sometimes, though not consistently; *rarely true* if their child exhibits the behavior rarely or only once in a while; and *not true* if their child does not exhibit the behavior.

Practitioners should encourage caregivers to carefully read each item and think about their child's behavior before selecting an answer. It may be necessary in some cases for a caregiver to observe a child before selecting a response to the item. For example, Item 8.3 on the Preschool Interval asks families to indicate whether "Child stays with motor activity for 10 minutes or longer" (see Figure 2.4). Caregivers may need to observe their child performing motor activities before selecting the appropriate response option.

Some local, regional, or state programs may require providers to track and report child progress over time, or some providers may wish to quantify progress in order to determine program or intervention effects. It is possible in these cases to assign numerical values to the SEAM response options, which, in turn, permits comparing and reporting on children's performance over successive assessment periods.

Numerical Scores   In order to examine the psychometric properties of the SEAM, it was necessary to assign numerical values to SEAM response options. The values for response options were as follows: *very true* = 3; *somewhat true* = 2; *rarely true* = 1; and *not true* = 0. Using these values permitted conducting psychometric analyses that are described in the Technical Report (see Chapter 7).

SEAM users may choose to use these numerical values to quantify item responses and summarize children's acquisition of skills in order to monitor child progress over time. It is important, however, that the user recognize that the application of these numerical values has not been empirically studied. No data have been gathered to indicate the validity of using these values to monitor child progress over time. The SEAM Summary Form on the CD-ROM (for print users) or as part of the PDF e-book (for digital users) provides a space for recording and summarizing item scores if programs choose to use numerical scores.

Concerns   In addition to scoring each item, caregivers should be directed to check the circle in the Concern column if the item is a concern for them. For example, the parents of a 20-month-old may mark Item 2.4 in the Toddler Interval (Toddler identifies her own emotions) as a concern because their toddler is not using words to indicate when he is angry, something his older sister did at that age (see Figure 2.5). Any item marked as a concern merits further discussion between the practitioner and the

		Very true	Somewhat true	Rarely true	Not true	Concern	Focus area
8.3	Child stays with motor activity for 10 minutes or longer.	☐	☑	☐	☐	○	△
	Some examples might be *Rides tricycle for 10 minutes* *Plays games such as Simon Says for 10 minutes*						

Figure 2.4.   Completed Item 8.3 from the Preschool Interval of the Social-Emotional Assessment/Evaluation Measure (SEAM™).

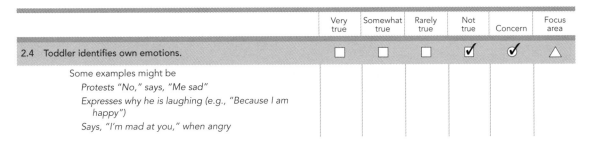

	Very true	Somewhat true	Rarely true	Not true	Concern	Focus area
2.4 Toddler identifies own emotions.	☐	☐	☐	☑	☑	△
Some examples might be *Protests "No," says, "Me sad"* *Expresses why he is laughing (e.g., "Because I am happy")* *Says, "I'm mad at you," when angry*						

Figure 2.5. Completed Item 2.4 from the Toddler Interval of the Social-Emotional Assessment/Evaluation Measure (SEAM™).

caregiver to determine the nature of the concern and whether additional follow-up may be necessary. If a concern does not warrant immediate follow-up, providers should periodically check in with caregivers to determine whether caregiver concerns about the skill have continued or increased; this can help caregivers and providers determine whether an item should become a focus area.

Focus Areas Finally, caregivers can check the triangle in the Focus Area column if they would like additional information, support, or resources in relation to the item or if they would like the item to become an intervention goal for their child. Practitioners and caregivers typically discuss whether an item should be a future focus area. For example, the parents previously mentioned may decide to mark Item 2.4 as a focus area for their toddler after discussing it with a practitioner to see whether he begins to use words to express his feelings after more focused assistance and support from them. Following is a suggestion of how a practitioner might explain the SEAM response options.

"After reading a SEAM item, consider the examples and think about your child's behavior before selecting an answer. You may want to observe your child before answering some of the questions. Remember, examples are there just to give you ideas about how the behavior might look. Your child may display the skills in a different way.

There are four options for rating your child's behavior. Select *very true* if your child does this skill or behavior consistently or most of the time. Select *somewhat true* if your child does this skill or behavior sometimes, though not consistently. Select *rarely true* if your child only does it once in a while, and *not true* if your child does not yet perform the skill.

Answer each question based on your experiences and what you know about your child. There is also a place for you to indicate if any particular item is a concern and another place to indicate if you would like an item to become a focus area that we work on with your child."

It is important for practitioners and caregivers to remember that behaviors may be displayed in different ways depending on a child's age, the developmental level of a child, and the expectations of culture and family. For example, Benchmark 7.0 on the Preschool Interval includes Item 7.1 (Child shows off work, takes pride in accomplishments). Although this behavior is considered developmentally appropriate for many families in the United States, it may not fit some families' cultural norms and expectations for their children and thus would not be an appropriate item to target as a focus area or goal.

As previously mentioned, each item is accompanied by several examples to give caregivers ideas about how the behavior might look. The way in which a child displays a behavior may or may not be illustrated by the corresponding examples. Caregivers may need guidance in some cases to determine whether the behaviors and skills their child demonstrates match the intent of particular items. In turn, the three SEAM intervals cover a wide range of development. Caregivers should understand that their particular child is not expected to do all of the behaviors on the SEAM. Questions can be omitted that do not seem relevant to the child at the time or appropriate for the family's values.

3

SEAM™ with Ages

The SEAM with Ages is available for the Infant, Toddler, and Preschool Intervals and parallels the SEAM. The only difference between the SEAM and the SEAM with Ages is that the latter includes corresponding age ranges for the examples provided with each item (see Figure 3.1).

The SEAM with Ages component is designed to assist practitioners in providing general guidance to caregivers about the ways in which children of different ages may be expected to exhibit target skills and behaviors. The ages were determined by using empirical data found in the literature and information from other existing tests. These age indices provide general guidelines and may not represent the skill ranges and variability of individual children. The SEAM with Ages can assist practitioners in understanding and explaining to caregivers the developmental progression of social-emotional skills and behaviors and where a child's development fits on the continuum of skill acquisition. The SEAM with Ages was *not* intended to be completed in addition to the SEAM. Practitioners may decide, however, to have some families complete the SEAM with Ages instead of the SEAM. For example, if a child is near age level in most skills and about to enter a community preschool, the family may want to know the skills and behaviors that are below age norms so that they can give the child the opportunity to practice these skills more in the home environment.

Average age in months		Very true	Somewhat true	Rarely true	Not true	Concern	Focus area
C-1.0 TODDLER PARTICIPATES IN HEALTHY INTERACTIONS							
1.1 Toddler lets you know if he needs help, attention, or comfort.		☐	☐	☐	☐	○	△
	Some examples might be						
18–24	Asks for a drink of water by pointing or showing you						
18–36	Pulls on you or other adult or raises arms to be picked up						
18–36	Goes to you or other familiar adults when hurt						
18–36	Seeks attention from you and other familiar adults; babbles and "shows off" for you						
24–36	Asks for a drink of water using one- or two-word utterances						
30–36	Calls for you when he needs help (e.g., "Daddy help")						
1.2 Toddler initiates and responds to affection.		☐	☐	☐	☐	○	△
	Some examples might be						
12–36	Comes when you ask or gesture for her to follow						
18–36	Hugs you; smiles back at you						
18–36	Hugs and kisses people, pets, and stuffed animals						
24–36	Returns hugs, kisses, or other affectionate gestures						
24–36	Walks to you with arms out, wanting a hug						
1.3 Toddler talks and plays with people whom he knows well.		☐	☐	☐	☐	○	△
	Some examples might be						
18–24	Points to show you things						
18–24	Begins to include you or siblings in play, pretends to offer you or others food, tries to care for baby sibling or dolls						
24–26	Uses one or two words to communicate with peers (e.g., "Car go?")						
24–36	Talks to you about his activities (e.g., "I push car")						
1.4 Toddler initiates and responds when you communicate with her.		☐	☐	☐	☐	○	△
	Some examples might be						
18–24	Answers your questions with one word (e.g., "juice")						
20–36	Asks questions (e.g., "Where mama?"), says, "Mama come" when she wants you to play						
30–36	Asks many questions (e.g., "Why?" "What?" "How?")						

Figure 3.1.   Sample from Benchmark 1.0 of the Toddler Interval of Social-Emotional Assessment/Evaluation Measure (SEAM™) with Ages.

4

SEAM™ Family Profile

The SEAM system includes a SEAM Family Profile assessment with intervals that correspond to the three SEAM intervals—Infant, Toddler, and Preschool. The cover sheets for each SEAM Family Profile assessment include the name of the interval (i.e., Infant, Toddler, Preschool) along with the developmental age range for each interval. As with the SEAM, a generic cover sheet is available that does not list the interval.

Each SEAM Family Profile interval is composed of four adult benchmarks with corresponding items to be assessed and scored. Benchmarks and corresponding items are designed to gather information about caregivers' strengths as well as the supports and resources they need to provide a safe, responsive, and emotionally nurturing environment for their children. The items focus on knowledge, skills, and resources that caregivers need in order to foster their child's social-emotional competence and are written in language that is easy to understand. Table 4.1 contains a list of Infant SEAM Family Profile benchmarks and items. A complete list of SEAM Family Profile benchmarks and items for all three intervals can be found in Appendix B.

Each family benchmark on the SEAM Family Profile is designated with an *F* and the associated benchmark number (e.g. F-1.0). Corresponding items are designated with the benchmark number followed by item number and separated by a period (e.g., 1.1, 1.2, 1.3). Figure 4.1 shows a sample benchmark from the Preschool Interval of the SEAM Family Profile with corresponding items and examples.

The number of items varies across benchmarks and intervals on the SEAM Family Profile. For example, Benchmark F-2.0 on the Toddler interval of the SEAM Family Profile (Providing activities that match my child's developmental level) has two corresponding items, whereas Benchmark F-1.0 on the Preschool Interval of the SEAM Family Profile (Responding to my preschooler's needs) has six corresponding items.

Each item is accompanied by several examples in order to assist caregivers in completing the SEAM Family Profile and give families ideas about how they might demonstrate the item. Item 2.1 from the Toddler Interval of the SEAM Family Profile (I provide my child books, toys, and playthings that match her developmental level) includes the following examples of how a caregiver might exhibit this item.

- I offer materials and toys that encourage her thinking and problem-solving skills, such as sorting toys into buckets, completing puzzles, and playing with puppets.

- I am able to provide toys and books that are safe and interesting to my child.

Table 4.1. Benchmarks and items from the Infant Interval of the Social-Emotional Assessment/Evaluation Measure (SEAM™) Family Profile

Benchmark	Item
F-1.0 Responding to my baby's needs	1.1 I understand my baby's nonverbal communication and know how to respond. 1.2 I understand my baby's verbal communication and know how to respond. 1.3 I know how to help my baby calm down.
F-2.0 Providing activities and playing with my baby	2.1 I provide books, toys, and playthings that are safe and that my baby enjoys. 2.2 I know games and activities that my baby enjoys.
F-3.0 Providing predictable schedule/routines and appropriate environment for my baby	3.1 I create and follow routines that make eating enjoyable and satisfying for me and my baby. 3.2 I provide a nap and sleeping schedule/routine for my baby that is predictable and appropriate for her age. 3.3 I use daily activities as playtime or make time each day to play with my baby.
F-4.0 Providing my baby with a safe home and play environment	4.1 I have done a safety check on my home to make it safe for my baby. 4.2 I have a safe way to transport my baby. 4.3 I know ways to keep my baby safe throughout the day. 4.4 I have someone I trust who can help take care of my baby. 4.5 I have access to health care for my baby. 4.6 I know how to manage feelings of anger or frustration that may occur while I am with my baby.

GUIDELINES FOR COMPLETING THE SEAM™ FAMILY PROFILE

The SEAM Family Profile can be completed in several ways. Whenever possible, practitioners should tailor caregiver participation to match the caregiver's individual needs and desires. They can provide caregivers with a copy of the SEAM Family Profile to independently complete, depending on their language and literacy level. They can also administer the SEAM Family Profile in the context of caregiver groups or classes, reviewing questions aloud as caregivers follow along and complete it. An interview format is the method of completion preferred by many practitioners because it allows them to clarify items, explain examples, explore concerns, and help caregivers choose appropriate response options. Items not relevant to caregivers can be omitted.

Introducing the SEAM™ Family Profile

It is ideal for a practitioner to have time to build a relationship with a caregiver and establish mutual trust and understanding before completing the SEAM Family Profile. The first step in completing the SEAM Family Profile is to explain to caregivers the purpose of the assessment. Following is an example of how a practitioner might introduce the SEAM Family Profile.

> "The SEAM Family Profile is designed to gather information about what you feel is going well in your relationship with your child as well as any supports and resources you might need to provide a safe and nurturing environment for your child. Items on the SEAM Family Profile focus on knowledge, skills, and resources caregivers need in order to foster their children's social-emotional development."

Scoring Guidelines for the SEAM™ Family Profile

Each SEAM Family Profile interval includes a cover sheet with space for entering identifying information and instructions for completion. Practitioners should read each item along with the examples after introducing the SEAM Family Profile and review item response options with caregivers. The cultural appropriateness of each item for individual families should be considered, and items that caregivers may find intrusive, disrespectful, or inappropriate should be omitted.

As shown in Figure 4.1, SEAM Family Profile intervals include three possible response options. For each item, caregivers can check the box under *most of the time* if the caregiver(s) feels he or she usually performs the skill or behavior described in the item. Caregivers can check *sometimes* if the caregiver(s) feels he or she only sometimes performs the skill or behavior described in the item. *Not yet* can be checked if the caregiver(s) feels he or she does not or is not able to perform the skill or behavior described in the item. Psychometric data have not been collected on the SEAM Family Profile, including the scoring options and their validity and reliability for identifying areas of competence and potential needs. Therefore, it is not recommended at this time to assign point values to responses on the SEAM Family Profile.

In addition to answering each item, caregivers should be directed to check the box under *not sure/ need more info* if they do not understand the item, are unsure of how to respond, or would like to get more information before choosing a final response option. Finally, caregivers should check the triangle in the Focus Area column if they need related resources or support (e.g., from child's teacher, home visitor, specialists) to better support their child's social-emotional development and well-being. Practitioners may assist parents in determining whether an item might be a future focus area.

Each item is accompanied by several examples to give caregivers ideas about how the behavior might look. A space is provided for caregivers to add their own examples. Following is a suggestion of how a practitioner might explain how to complete the SEAM Family Profile.

"After reading a SEAM Family Profile item, consider the examples and think about your family and relationship with your child before selecting an answer. Examples are offered as ideas about how your family's interactions with your child might look. You and other family members may have different ways that you demonstrate these items; there is space for you to write in your own examples.

There are three response options for each item. Check the box under *most of the time* if you usually perform the skill or behavior described in the item. Check *sometimes* if you only sometimes perform the skill or behavior. Check *not yet* if you do not or are not able to perform the skill or behavior.

Answer based on your personal experiences and what you feel is true for you. There is also a place for you to indicate if you do not understand the item, are unsure of how to respond, or would like to get more information before choosing a response option. There is another place to indicate if you would like an item to become a focus area. This means you might like some resources, support, or information from a professional to help you with this item."

	Most of the time	Sometimes	Not yet	Not sure/ need more info	Focus area
F-3.0 PROVIDING PREDICTABLE SCHEDULE/ROUTINES AND APPROPRIATE ENVIRONMENT FOR MY CHILD					
3.1 I provide a mealtime routine for my child that is predictable and appropriate for his age.	☐	☐	☐	☐	△

Some examples might be

I provide my child with meals and snacks at regular times each day.

I include my child in meal preparation when possible (e.g., picking out vegetables, measuring and stirring, helping set the table).

Please give examples of foods you provide and your mealtime routine:

	Most of the time	Sometimes	Not yet	Not sure/ need more info	Focus area
3.2 I provide a rest and sleeping routine for my child that is predictable and appropriate for her age.	☐	☐	☐	☐	△

Some examples might be

I provide bedtime and naptime at consistent times across days and weeks.

I help my child follow a simple routine before bed (e.g., taking a bath, brushing teeth, taking time to quietly read books together).

Please give examples of your child's naptime and bedtime routines:

	Most of the time	Sometimes	Not yet	Not sure/ need more info	Focus area
3.3 I provide my child with predictable limits and consequences.	☐	☐	☐	☐	△

Some examples might be

I provide my child with consistent limits and rules (e.g., no hitting or running in the house).

I notice and comment to my child when he is doing something positive and consistent with our household rules (e.g., "I like the way you are putting away your clothes")

Please give examples of how you provide predictable limits and consequences for your child:

	Most of the time	Sometimes	Not yet	Not sure/ need more info	Focus area
3.4 I take time each day to play with my child.	☐	☐	☐	☐	△

Some examples might be

I take time each day to laugh and be silly with my child.

I play rhyming games and sing songs with my child as we go through the day.

Please give examples of times of day when you play with your child and playful activities you do together:

Figure 4.1.   Sample from Benchmark F-3.0 of the Preschool Interval of the Social-Emotional Assessment/Evaluation Measure (SEAM™) Family Profile.

5

Summarizing SEAM™ Information

Reviewing and summarizing the information gathered from the completed SEAM and SEAM Family Profile is the final step of the assessment process. The practitioner should review the information from both assessments and clarify any discrepancies or questions with the caregiver(s). For example, if a home visitor notes that a child has difficulty regulating her emotional responses during home visits but her mother indicates on the SEAM that the child is able to consistently perform this skill, then a discussion should ensue to help both parties understand this difference in their perceptions and determine whether the item should be a focus area. Practitioners can then provide families with activities that support the child's and family's development of selected skills and guide caregivers in providing children with opportunities to practice these skills within the context of daily family routines and activities.

Once SEAM measures are completed and questions and inconsistencies are resolved, the next step is to summarize and integrate the information from the SEAM and SEAM Family Profile. The SEAM Summary Form provided for each SEAM interval permits summarizing child and family strengths, family concerns, and items selected as focus areas based on information gathered when completing the SEAM and the SEAM Family Profile (see Figure 5.1).

The first section of the SEAM Summary Form provides space for recording SEAM assessment information and indicating whether each item is a child's strength, a concern for the family that needs monitoring, or an agreed-on focus area. The form also contains a column in which professionals can record numerical item scores as well as a place for recording a total numerical score if that option is chosen. As previously mentioned, numerical scores may assist professionals in quantifying item responses, summarizing children's acquisition of skills, and monitoring child progress over time. These applications have not been empirically verified, however. No data have been gathered to date to indicate how the SEAM functions in terms of monitoring child progress over time.

The second section of the SEAM Summary Form provides space for recording information gathered through the SEAM Family Profile. This form includes columns for indicating whether an item is a family strength, the family needs additional information about the item, or the item is an agreed-on focus area. Both sections of the Summary Form allow practitioners to record results for three separate assessment periods. As previously mentioned, the SEAM Family Profile does not include space for recording scores because numerical values have not yet been assigned to the response options.

SEAM Social-Emotional Assessment/ Evaluation Measure RESEARCH EDITION

Summary Form
Infant
for developmental range 2–18 months

Child's name: ______________________________

Adult/caregiver's name: ______________________________

INSTRUCTIONS: The SEAM (C) and SEAM Family Profile (F) benchmarks and their associated items are listed on the following pages. Beside each item is space to enter the administration date and whether the item has been identified as a strength (i.e., as indicated by checking *very true* on an item on the SEAM and *most of the time* on an item on the SEAM Family Profile). There is also space to indicate whether an item is a concern and needs monitoring (i.e., as indicated by a check in the circle in the Concern column) or whether the item has been selected as a focus area (as indicated by a check in the triangle for the Focus area column). The form can be used to enter data from three separate administrations.

	Admin date:________				Admin date:________				Admin date:________			
SEAM	Strength	Concern/continue monitoring	Focus area	Numerical score (optional)	Strength	Concern/continue monitoring	Focus area	Numerical score (optional)	Strength	Concern/continue monitoring	Focus area	Numerical score (optional)
Benchmark C-1.0												
Item 1.1												
Item 1.2												
Item 1.3												
Item 1.4												
Benchmark C-2.0												
Item 2.1												
Item 2.2												
Item 2.3												
Benchmark C-3.0												
Item 3.1												
Item 3.2												
Item 3.3												
Benchmark C-4.0												
Item 4.1												
Item 4.2												
Item 4.3												
Item 4.4												

Figure 5.1. Excerpt from the Infant Interval of the Social-Emotional Assessment/Evaluation Measure (SEAM™) Summary Form.

SEAM assessment information can be used to develop individualized family service plan (IFSP) or individualized education program (IEP) goals and family outcomes. SEAM results can be formulated into objective, measureable goals or objectives that can be directly incorporated into intervention plans for children.

6

Scenario
Using the SEAM™ and the SEAM™ Family Profile

The following scenario provides an illustration of how caregivers and practitioners might collaborate in using the SEAM system to assess a child and family and plan for subsequent intervention efforts based on SEAM results.

Sunshine Center is a neighborhood early child care facility that supports the education and general development of toddlers. The mission of the Sunshine Center includes a commitment to helping children develop positive social-emotional competence. In support of this mission, all caregivers complete a social-emotional assessment—the SEAM—at regular intervals while their children are enrolled at the Sunshine Center.

Maria and Samuel have a 2-year-old daughter, Rose, who attends the Sunshine Center; her teacher is Ms. Sanchez. After getting to know Rose and her parents, Ms. Sanchez visits their home to complete the Toddler Interval of the SEAM. She plans to ask them later to complete the SEAM Family Profile. Rose's parents are offered several alternative methods for completing the SEAM, and they select the interview option. Ms. Sanchez reads each item and some of the examples while Maria and Samuel read along from their copy of the SEAM protocol. Maria and Samuel indicate the response option for each item that best represents Rose's behavior (e.g., *very true*).

When Ms. Sanchez asks about Rose's ability "to settle herself down after periods of exciting activity" (Item 3.2), Maria describes the family ritual of after-dinner playtime when Rose and Samuel wrestle and play chase together. Although this activity takes place well before bedtime, Rose often has difficulty calming down afterward and "falling asleep without a problem" (Item 10.3). Bedtime has become a long, drawn-out, and frustrating process. Rose's parents agree that this is a concern, and they want to know how to help Rose calm down. Figure 6.1 shows how Rose's parents completed Item 3.2 on the Toddler Interval of the SEAM.

Ms. Sanchez and Rose's parents agree to focus on helping Rose settle down following vigorous play. Ms. Sanchez agrees to provide classroom strategies designed to help all children in her classroom calm down after exciting activities and make the transition into new ones. She also helps Maria and

				Very true	Somewhat true	Rarely true	Not true	Concern	Focus area
3.2	Toddler can settle self down after periods of exciting activity.			☐	☐	☑	☐	○	◬
	Some examples might be								
	Calms self with your help after a game of chase								
	Sits down and calms self after an exciting activity								

Figure 6.1. Item 3.2 of the Toddler Interval of the Social-Emotional Assessment Evaluation Measure (SEAM™) completed for Rose.

Samuel create strategies to help Rose get to sleep at night. Ms. Sanchez gives Maria and Samuel the Toddler Interval of the SEAM Family Profile to complete and review at a later time.

During the weeks following her initial meeting with Rose's parents, Ms. Sanchez monitors Rose's progress at calming down following exciting or stimulating activities during the day. Maria and Samuel monitor Rose's progress at home before bedtime.

Ms. Sanchez and Rose's parents compare notes at their next home visit and agree that Rose's ability to calm down before bed has improved somewhat, but they decide to continue working on this goal with her. Samuel and Maria also identify a second focus area, indicating that Rose does not consistently "accept changes in routines and settings" (Item 10.2). In fact, at home Rose often cries and becomes frustrated when asked to stop one activity and begin another. It is difficult to leave the house to go somewhere, and Rose's parents do not understand what she wants and why she is upset. Ms. Sanchez has also noticed that Rose continues to struggle with making transitions between classroom activities.

In addition, Ms. Sanchez and Rose's parents review the completed SEAM Family Profile. Maria and Samuel have checked *sometimes* for the following: "I understand my child's nonverbal communication and know how to respond" (Item 1.1), "I know how to successfully redirect my child's inappropriate behaviors" (Item 1.5) and "I understand why my child engages in inappropriate behaviors and know how to modify the environment" (Item 1.6). Maria and Samuel checked the Focus Area triangle for all three of these items to indicate that they would like them to be areas of focus in their work with Rose. They also checked *sometimes* for "I provide my child with predictable limits and consequences" (Item 3.3), and they say they would like this to be a focus area as well. Figure 6.2 shows Items 1.4, 1.5, and 1.6 from the Toddler Interval of the SEAM Family Profile completed by Maria and Samuel.

Maria and Samuel indicate at the conclusion of the meeting that they would like to keep working on Rose's ability to calm herself and to make transitions, as well as to work on understanding and redirecting Rose's inappropriate behavior and modifying their home environment in ways that will support positive behaviors and successful transitions. Maria, Samuel, and Ms. Sanchez develop a plan together to address these concerns. Ms. Sanchez agrees to focus on communication and social-emotional skill building with her class. Maria and Samuel thank Ms. Sanchez for acknowledging their concerns, validating their feelings, and working on these issues together. They express their enthusiasm and hope that with additional support Rose will be less frustrated and more able to communicate with them about her wants and needs.

	Most of the time	Sometimes	Not yet	Not sure/ need more info	Focus area
1.4 I use positive comments and language with my child.	☑	☐	☐	☐	△

Some examples might be

I comment on how gentle my child is being when he is petting the cat.

I give my child a high-five when he picks up his toys.

Please give examples of positive language you use and comments you say to your child:

I often tell Emma, "You did it!" when she has done something like putting on her shoes or her coat all by herself.

	Most of the time	Sometimes	Not yet	Not sure/ need more info	Focus area
1.5 I know how to successfully redirect my child's inappropriate behaviors.	☐	☑	☐	☐	☑

Some examples might be

I give my child her favorite doll before she pokes her baby sister.

I remind my child to walk indoors when she begins to run, or I take her outside to play.

Please give examples of ways you redirect your child's inappropriate behaviors:

When Emma does something naughty, I usually tell her, "That's not okay," and pick her up and move her, but sometimes it doesn't work. It makes her mad.

	Most of the time	Sometimes	Not yet	Not sure/ need more info	Focus area
1.6 I understand why my child engages in inappropriate behaviors and know how to modify the environment.	☐	☑	☐	☐	☑

Some examples might be

I prepare my child for a long bus ride by providing him with art and other enjoyable activities to keep him occupied during the trip.

I let my child choose one grocery item at the store before a tantrum occurs.

Please give examples of ways that you prevent inappropriate behaviors:

When Emma cries and doesn't want to go to bed, I think she is scared, so I turn on a light for her. Sometimes she will go to sleep, but other times she keeps crying, and I don't know what to do for her.

Figure 6.2. Items 1.4–1.6 of the Toddler Interval of the Social-Emotional Assessment Evaluation Measure (SEAM™) Family Profile completed by Rose's parents, Maria and Samuel.

7

Technical Report

The SEAM was developed to address the need for psychometrically sound social-emotional assessment tools for young children. The SEAM was designed as a curriculum-based assessment measure to assist in the prevention and early identification of social-emotional difficulties and behavior disorders, as well as to build positive partnerships with families and optimize positive caregiver–child interactions in the first years of life.

SEAM benchmarks and items were identified from the literature on social-emotional development of young children raised in mainly Western cultures; certain concepts repeatedly emerged as those that were deemed essential or critically important to the mental health competence of young children (Squires & Bricker, 2007). These benchmarks and items were reviewed and revised in an iterative process based on feedback from family members and experts in infant mental health, early childhood, early intervention/early childhood special education, psychology, and behavior disorders. Any items that appeared difficult to understand or with ambiguous meanings were revised based on expert and caregiver feedback.

The psychometric properties of the SEAM were investigated in a series of research studies that are reported in this chapter. Psychometric studies on the Infant and Toddler Intervals were conducted as part of a federally funded research grant; pencil-and-paper as well as online data were gathered from a variety of caregivers served in programs around the United States. Additional data were also collected on Infant, Toddler, and Preschool Intervals through an online research web site (Squires et al., 2012a, 2012b). Research questions included the following:

- What is the item functioning for the Infant and Toddler Intervals?

- What is the reliability of the Infant, Toddler, and Preschool Intervals, including internal consistency, test–retest, and interrater reliability?

- What is the validity of the Infant, Toddler, and Preschool Intervals, specifically content and congruent validity?

- What is the utility of the SEAM system as rated by caregivers and early interventionists?

SAMPLE

The pencil-and-paper data were gathered from caregivers and practitioners in early childhood programs serving typically developing children and children with developmental delays. Online data were gathered from a variety of caregivers around the United States using a research web site. Paper-and-pencil data, including demographic and utility surveys, were completed one of several ways, including individually by caregivers without practitioner assistance, by caregivers during an interview with a practitioner, and by a practitioner with at least 20 hours of weekly contact with a child (for interrater reliability). Practitioners included 1) early childhood classroom teachers and assistants primarily working with infants and toddlers who were typically developing and 2) early interventionists/early childhood special educators working with families and their children who were at risk or eligible for Part C services. Online measures, including demographic and utility surveys as well as SEAM intervals, were independently completed by caregivers, for the most part without assistance.

Data were collected in 49 states across the United States and from Canada. The number of completed SEAMs from each state ranged from 1 to 279, with the largest number coming from Oregon. The sample included a total of 2,201 SEAMs; 1,850 were collected online, and 351 were collected from paper-and-pencil versions. Of the sample, 59% of children were male and 41% were female. The children represented in the sample were predominately Caucasian (76.1%). Other ethnicities included multiracial (6.2%), Hispanic/Latino (4.9%), African American (4.7%), Asian (3.7%), American Indian/Alaskan Native (1.1%), Native Hawaiian/Pacific Islander (0.1%), other nonspecified ethnicity (1.4%), and unknown (1.8%). Fifty-eight percent of children were typically developing, whereas 42% of children were identified with a disability or developmental delay.

Data on family income and education level also were collected. The majority of caregivers reported incomes greater than $50,000 (57%), whereas 43% reported incomes below that level. The greatest percentage of participating caregivers (60%) had a bachelor's or postgraduate/graduate degree, whereas 19% had some college, 17% had a high school diploma or general equivalency diploma, and 4% had not completed high school.

Data analysis techniques included item response theory (IRT) modeling as well as classical test analyses. IRT modeling was used to examine item order and fit statistics while traditional test analyses were employed to complete validity and reliability studies.

PENCIL-AND-PAPER AND ONLINE DATA COLLECTION

Before proceeding to data analysis, a differential item functioning (DIF) analysis using a Rasch one parameter logistic (1PL) partial credit model (PCM) for polytomous scoring (Masters & Wright, 1997) was completed with the estimation software Winsteps 3.73 (Linacre, 2011) in order to examine whether SEAM items appeared to be functioning differently with different administration methods (i.e., paper/pencil and online) for the Infant and Toddler Intervals. The results from the DIF analysis indicated that there were only minor differences in item functioning between administration methods. Evidence for significant DIF was demonstrated in 3 out of 35 items (8.6%) in the Infant Interval and 2 out of 35 items (5.7%) in the Toddler Interval. These results suggested that most of the items functioned invariantly and were not affected by extraneous artifacts inherent in the method of completion by the rater. Similar results were found for ability status; 5 out of 35 items (14.3%) demonstrated DIF on the Infant Interval, whereas only 2 out of 35 items (5.7%) on the Toddler Interval had evidence of significant DIF. These results suggested minimal bias between groups. These findings supported the rationale for analyzing the data set as a whole.

QUESTION 1: WHAT IS THE ITEM FUNCTIONING FOR THE INFANT AND TODDLER SEAM™ INTERVALS?

Item Fit Statistics

Item fit statistics are generated as an indication of how well the selected model (i.e., Rasch 1PL PCM) fits the obtained data. Responses to items from people of varying estimated abilities should be consistent with the estimated item difficulty, such that participants with estimated high ability should·be

Table 7.1. Item fit statistics

Age interval	Benchmark	Infit mean MNSQ (*SD*)	Infit MNSQ range	Outfit mean MNSQ (*SD*)	Outfit MNSQ range	Item ordering
Infant	1.0	0.98 (0.19)	0.84–1.29	0.95 (0.17)	0.81–1.23	*a, d, b, c*
	2.0	0.97 (0.21)	0.79–1.26	0.97 (0.24)	0.71–1.29	a, b, c
	3.0	0.99 (0.08)	0.89–1.09	0.97 (0.05)	0.89–1.02	b, a, c
	4.0	0.99 (0.10)	0.87–1.14	0.93 (0.14)	0.78–1.16	*b, c, d, a*
	5.0	1.00 (0.28)	0.74–1.44	1.16 (0.52)	0.74–*2.01*	b, a, c, d
	6.0	0.95 (0.16)	0.73–1.17	1.14 (0.31)	0.79–1.45	b, a, c, d
	7.0	1.00 (0.12)	0.87–1.16	0.95 (0.11)	0.84–1.10	*c, a, b*
	8.0	0.98 (0.09)	0.86–1.08	1.01 (0.14)	0.82–1.11	a, c, b
	9.0	1.00 (0.06)	0.92–1.06	0.92 (0.04)	0.87–0.97	a, b, c
	10.0	1.00 (0.11)	0.87–1.16	0.94 (0.15)	0.73–1.11	*d, a, c, b*
Toddler	1.0	1.00 (0.22)	0.73–1.23	1.00 (0.23)	0.74–1.25	*d, b, a, c*
	2.0	1.02 (0.26)	0.68–1.35	*2.70 (3.12)*	0.69–*8.09*	a, b, c, d
	3.0	0.99 (0.13)	0.84–1.17	1.03 (0.17)	0.84–1.25	a, b, c
	4.0	0.97 (0.12)	0.85–1.14	0.99 (0.12)	0.89–1.16	a, b, c
	5.0	0.99 (0.05)	0.92–1.06	1.00 (0.07)	0.92–1.08	b, a, c, e, d
	6.0	1.00 (0.06)	0.95–1.08	0.98 (0.04)	0.95–1.04	*c, b, a*
	7.0	0.98 (0.13)	0.83–1.14	0.98 (0.16)	0.79–1.19	a, c, b
	8.0	0.99 (0.11)	0.88–1.15	0.98 (0.12)	0.85–1.15	*c, d, a, b*
	9.0	0.98 (0.05)	0.94–1.03	0.93 (0.02)	0.92–0.95	a, b
	10.0	1.00 (0.10)	0.87–1.15	0.99 (0.12)	0.85–1.17	a, c, b, d
Preschool	1.0	0.99 (0.14)	0.76–1.17	0.92 (0.18)	0.65–1.20	*a, b, c, e, d*
	2.0	0.98 (0.14)	0.85–1.20	1.25 (0.43)	0.84–1.88	a, b, c, d
	3.0	0.99 (0.13)	0.83–1.20	0.97 (0.15)	0.79–1.15	*c, a, b, d*
	4.0	0.98 (0.04)	0.94–1.02	0.98 (0.04)	0.93–1.02	a, b
	5.0	0.99 (0.14)	0.80–1.18	1.00 (0.16)	0.80–1.24	*a, b, d, c*
	6.0	0.99 (0.15)	0.85–1.25	1.00 (0.21)	0.80–1.36	*a, d, b, c*
	7.0	0.98 (0.21)	0.80–1.28	0.94 (0.21)	0.78–1.24	*b, c, a*
	8.0	0.99 (0.13)	0.83–1.16	0.99 (0.16)	0.80–1.23	*e, b, a, c, d*
	9.0	0.99 (0.05)	0.93–1.05	0.93 (0.05)	0.87–0.99	*b, a, c*
	10.0	1.00 (0.12)	0.85–1.22	0.96 (0.14)	0.77–1.21	*g, e, f, a, b, d, c*

Letters are used instead of numbers for item ordering to facilitate visual analysis of the results (e.g., a = 1.1, b = 1.2, c = 1.3, d = 1.4, e = 1.5, f = 1.6, g = 1.7 for Preschool Benchmark 1.0). Italicized and bolded value indicates a misfit detected.
Key: MNSQ, mean square; SD, standard deviation.

able to demonstrate more difficult skills, whereas participants with lower ability should only be able to do easier items. Items that fit the model well are assigned fit statistics that range in value from 0.5 to 1.5. Items less than 0.5 are considered overly predictive, whereas items that are greater than 1.5 contain more noise than useful information and are considered degrading to the measure (Linacre, 2011). Confirming adequate model fit is a necessary step for ensuring credibility of results when performing an IRT modeling analysis. We examined item fit (i.e., outfit mean square) within each SEAM benchmark for this analysis. Results indicated that item-level fit statistics were well within the acceptable range for the majority of benchmarks, except for Item 5.1 (fit statistics = 2.01) from Benchmark 5.0 in the Infant Interval, Item 2.1 (fit statistics = 8.09) from Benchmark 2.0 in the Toddler Interval, and Item 2.1 (fit statistics = 1.88) from Benchmark 2.0 in the Preschool Interval (see Table 7.1). These results provide evidence of unidimensionality for each benchmark and support the use of the Rasch 1PL PCM as a means to evaluate item functioning.

Item Functioning

Item functioning was evaluated in order to better understand the contribution of individual items within each benchmark of the SEAM. As previously mentioned, IRT offers a range of latent trait measurement models for explaining the relation between item responses and two classes of unobserved variables: 1) person ability and 2) item characteristics (Embretson & Reise, 2000; Hambleton & Swaminathan, 1985). Item characteristics (e.g., difficulty, sensitivity) are estimated with the person's responses to the set of measurement items, and each person's ability level is estimated based on his or her set of responses and the estimated item characteristics.

One of the purposes for doing the IRT modeling analysis was to examine the ordering of the items within each benchmark. Items within benchmarks on the experimental version of the SEAM

Table 7.2. Item functioning and Social-Emotional Assessment/Evaluation Measure (SEAM™) benchmarks with item order changes

Age interval	Benchmark			Original order and wording	Order from IRT modeling analysis	Final order
Infant	C-1.0	Baby participates in healthy interactions.	1.1	Baby shows interest in you and other familiar caregivers.	1.1	1.1
			1.2	Baby responds to you and other familiar caregivers.	1.4	1.3
			1.3	Baby initiates and responds to communications.	1.2	1.4
			1.4	Baby lets you know if she needs help or comfort.	1.3	1.2
	C-4.0	Baby begins to show empathy for others.	4.1	Baby mimics your facial expressions.	4.2	4.1
			4.2	Baby looks at and notices you and other familiar caregivers.	4.3	4.2
			4.3	Baby looks at and notices others' emotional responses.	4.4	4.3
			4.4	Baby responds to another's distress, seeking comfort for self.	4.1	4.4
	C-7.0	Baby displays a positive self-image.	7.1	Baby laughs at, or smiles at, her image or picture of self.	7.3	7.2
			7.2	Baby recognizes his name.	7.1	7.3
			7.3	Baby calls attention to herself.	7.2	7.1
	C-10.0	Baby shows a range of adaptive skills.	10.1	Baby eats and gains weight on schedule.	10.4	10.2
			10.2	Baby eats a variety of age-appropriate foods.	10.1	10.4
			10.3	Baby sleeps with few problems.	10.3	10.3
			10.4	Baby eliminates (pees and poops) on regular schedule.	10.2	10.1
Toddler	C-1.0	Participates in healthy interactions	1.1	Toddler talks and plays with people whom she knows well.	1.4	1.3
			1.2	Toddler initiates and responds to affection.	1.2	1.2
			1.3	Toddler initiates and responds when you communicate with her.	1.1	1.4
			1.4	Toddler lets you know if he needs help, attention, or comfort.	1.3	1.1
	C-6.0	Demonstrates independence	6.1	Toddler explores new environments, while maintaining some contact.	6.3	6.3
			6.2	Toddler can separate from you in familiar environment with minimal distress.	6.2	6.2
			6.3	Toddler tries new tasks before seeking help.	6.1	6.1
	C-8.0	Regulates attention and activity level	8.1	Toddler stays with motor activities for 5 minutes or longer.	8.3	8.3
			8.2	Toddler looks at book or listens to a story for 5 minutes or longer.	8.4	8.4
			8.3	Toddler moves from one activity to another without problems.	8.1	8.1
			8.4	Toddler participates in simple games.	8.2	8.2
Preschool	C-3.0	Regulates social emotional responses	3.1	Child responds to peer's or caregiver's soothing when upset.	3.3	3.2
			3.2	Child can calm self when upset within 5 minutes.	3.1	3.3
			3.3	Child can calm self after periods of exciting activity.	3.2	3.1
			3.4	Child remains calm in disappointing situations.	3.4	3.4
	C-6.0	Demonstrates independence	6.1	Child explores new materials and settings.	6.1	6.1
			6.2	Child tries new task before seeking help.	6.4	6.3
			6.3	Child stays with or returns to challenging activities.	6.2	6.4
			6.4	Child can leave you without distress.	6.3	6.2
	C-7.0	Displays positive self-image	7.1	Child knows personal information.	7.2	7.3
			7.2	Child shows off work, takes pride in accomplishments.	7.3	7.1
			7.3	Child makes positive statements about self.	7.1	7.2
	C-8.0	Regulates attention and activity level	8.1	Child stays with motor activity for 10 minutes or longer.	8.5	8.3
			8.2	Child participates in early literacy activities.	8.2	8.2
			8.3	Child moves from one activity to another without problems.	8.1	8.4
			8.4	Child participates in games with others.	8.3	8.5
			8.5	Child regulates his activity level to match setting.	8.4	8.1
	C-10.0	Shows a range of adaptive skills	10.1	Child feeds self and eats a variety of foods without a problem.	10.7	10.4
			10.2	Child dresses self.	10.5	10.5
			10.3	Child goes to bed and falls asleep without a problem.	10.6	10.7
			10.4	Child uses the toilet appropriately.	10.1	10.6
			10.5	Child manages changes in settings and conditions.	10.2	10.2
			10.6	Child keeps himself safe in potentially dangerous conditions.	10.4	10.3
			10.7	Child solves problems to meet her needs.	10.3	10.1

Key: IRT, item response theory.

were intended to be ordered from easier to more difficult to facilitate an examination of a child's progress in social-emotional competencies. This initial item ordering was based on developmental quotient, or the relative difficulty of skills from the literature on social-emotional development of young children. Results from the estimated item difficulty suggested that the majority of items within each SEAM benchmark were in fact hierarchically organized (i.e., the numerical order reflects the developmental hierarchy of items, with "x.1" as the easiest) and confirmed the predetermined developmental hierarchy of these social-emotional skills (see Table 7.1). Benchmarks remained in the predetermined item order when only minor item order changes were indicated (e.g., switching the order of two adjacent items). The item order within four benchmarks on the Infant Interval, three benchmarks in the Toddler Interval, and five benchmarks in the Preschool Interval was found to be largely different from the hypothesized order (see Table 7.2). According to the IRT modeling analysis of item responses, the preidentified easier or easiest item within these benchmarks was, in fact, more difficult or in some cases appeared to be the most difficult item. Researchers considered the IRT suggested ordering of items for the benchmarks in which misorder was detected and carefully examined each set of items to determine whether the disagreement appeared to be due to 1) true item misorder or 2) misinterpretation of the item by respondents. The decision was then made to either reorder the items as suggested by the IRT results or to keep the items in their original position. Items were reordered according to the IRT results in most cases; however, original item ordering was maintained for a few benchmarks, and minor editing was done (either to the item itself, its accompanying example[s], or both) in an attempt to increase the clarity of individual items.

QUESTION 2: WHAT IS THE RELIABILITY OF THE INFANT, TODDLER, AND PRESCHOOL SEAM™ INTERVALS, INCLUDING INTERNAL CONSISTENCY, TEST–RETEST, AND INTER-RATER RELIABILITY?

Interrater Reliability

Interrater reliability data for the Infant and Toddler Intervals were collected from teacher dyads working at a high-quality child care center serving primarily children of University of Oregon faculty and staff. Master teachers and assistant teachers from the infant and toddler classrooms participated. Pearson product moment correlation coefficients and intraclass correlations were computed to examine interrater agreement. Results are presented in Table 7.3 for four teacher dyads (one dyad for the Infant Interval of the SEAM, $n = 12$ children) and three dyads for the Toddler Interval of the SEAM (Toddler Class 1, $n = 7$ children; Toddler Class 2, $n = 7$ children; and Toddler Class 3, $n = 8$ children). The Pearson product moment correlation coefficient ($r = .776$) was significant at $p < .01$ for the Infant Interval of the SEAM. The Pearson product moment correlation coefficient for Toddler Class 2 ($r = .948$) was also significant at $p < .01$. Pearson product moment correlation coefficients for Toddler Classes 1 and 3 were not significant. Intraclass correlations were also analyzed to examine the consistency of differences between scores across raters. Results of the intraclass correlations were strong and significant for teachers in the infant classroom and for toddler teachers in Classes 1 and 2, but were not significant for the teachers in Toddler Class 3 (see Table 7.3).

Test–Retest Reliability

Test–retest reliability data were collected by online caregiver participants. After completing the SEAM via a research web site, caregivers were immediately given the option to complete a second SEAM,

Table 7.3. Correlations of total Social-Emotional Assessment/Evaluation Measure (SEAM™) scores between professional raters within classrooms

Classroom	n	r	Intraclass correlation
Infant 1	12	.776**	.564*
Toddler 1	7	.668	.657*
Toddler 2	7	.948**	.932**
Toddler 3	8	.640	.324

Key: *p < .05; **p < .01.

Squires et al.

Table 7.4. Test–retest correlations

SEAM™ interval	n	r
Infant	43	.987**
Toddler	42	.968**
Preschool	49	.989**

Key: *p < .05; **p < .01; SEAM™; Social-Emotional Assessment/ Evaluation Measure.

Table 7.5. Correlations between Infant Social-Emotional Assessment/Evaluation Measure (SEAM™) benchmarks and overall SEAM scores

Benchmark	1	2	3	4	5	6	7	8	9	Total score
1.0										.85
2.0	.65									.83
3.0	.40	.36								.73
4.0	.66	.59	.42							.84
5.0	.62	.56	.36	.67						.85
6.0	.41	.56	.28	.47	.53					.82
7.0	.58	.59	.32	.62	.67	.65				.83
8.0	.55	.55	.35	.58	.64	.63	.67			.83
9.0	.36	.31	.37	.37	.36	.30	.31	.42		.69
10.0	.35	.31	.49	.36	.41	.44	.43	.44	.41	.77

Note: All correlations are significant at *p* < .01. Total number of Infant SEAMs included in the analyses between benchmarks ranged from 1,130 to 1,134 and was 1,153 for benchmark correlations with SEAM total score.

Table 7.6. Correlations between Toddler Social-Emotional Assessment/Evaluation Measure (SEAM™) benchmarks and overall SEAM scores

Benchmark	1	2	3	4	5	6	7	8	9	Total score
1.0										.87
2.0	.54									.84
3.0	.35	.32								.78
4.0	.56	.66	.33							.82
5.0	.62	.43	.41	.58						.90
6.0	.42	.36	.43	.44	.63					.82
7.0	.59	.65	.31	.68	.56	.43				.79
8.0	.49	.45	.51	.49	.62	.58	.55			.88
9.0	.51	.39	.42	.48	.62	.49	.58	.59		.84
10.0	.45	.46	.49	.50	.47	.47	.53	.51	.53	.83

Note: All correlations are significant at *p* < .01. Total number of Toddler SEAMs included in the analyses between benchmarks ranged from 467 to 472 and was 490 for benchmark correlations with SEAM total score.

blind to the results of the first one. Results indicated strong, significant agreement between the two SEAM completions for all three intervals (see Table 7.4).

Internal Consistency

Internal consistency of the SEAM was addressed by examining the relation between average benchmark scores using correlational analyses and Cronbach's coefficient alpha (Cronbach, 1951). Pearson product moment correlation coefficients between benchmarks ranged from .28 to .67 for the Infant Interval of the SEAM, from .31 to .68 for the Toddler Interval of the SEAM, and from .41 to .81 for the Preschool Interval of the SEAM (see Tables 7.5, 7.6, and 7.7). In addition, the correlational analyses between benchmarks and overall SEAM scores were consistent, ranging from .69 to .85 for the Infant Interval, from .78 to .90 for the Toddler Interval, and from .73 to .88 for the Preschool Interval. All correlations were significant, suggesting congruence between benchmarks within each age interval as well as between benchmarks and total SEAM scores. Cronbach's coefficient alphas were also calculated for each age interval. The standardized alpha was .90 for the Infant Interval, .91 for the Toddler Interval, and .96 for the Preschool Interval, indicating strong internal consistency.

Table 7.7. Correlations between Preschool Social-Emotional Assessment/Evaluation Measure (SEAM™) benchmarks and overall SEAM scores

Benchmark	1	2	3	4	5	6	7	8	9	Total score
1.0										.88
2.0	.76									.78
3.0	.60	.47								.74
4.0	.74	.69	.56							.78
5.0	.81	.67	.57	.70						.87
6.0	.61	.51	.50	.51	.58					.73
7.0	.69	.67	.41	.55	.65	.52				.76
8.0	.73	.61	.64	.64	.75	.60	.64			.88
9.0	.62	.49	.63	.54	.62	.47	.52	.71		.78
10.0	.61	.55	.61	.52	.60	.59	.55	.73	.66	.84

Note: All correlations are significant at $p < .01$. Total number of Preschool SEAMs included in the analyses between benchmarks ranged from 604 to 653 and was 524 for benchmark correlations with SEAM total score.

Table 7.8. Mean Social-Emotional Assessment/Evaluation Measure (SEAM™) scores and correlations with age across 6-month intervals

Age in months	n	M	r
SEAM for Infants	235		.354**
0–6	49	84.32	
6–12	153	93.49	
12–18	33	97.61	
SEAM for Toddlers	56		.391**
18–24	20	82.39	
24–30	19	86.83	
30–36	17	92.59	
SEAM for Preschool	240		.124
36–42	79	103.82	
42–48	62	107.89	
48–54	53	106.42	
54–60	35	108.49	
60–66	11	106.91	

Key: $^*p < .05$; $^{**}p < .01$.
Note: Age ranges begin on the first day of the first month indicated and end the day before the last month indicated. For example, the 6–12 month age range includes children who are between 6 months, 0 days old and 11 months and 30/31 days old.

QUESTION 3: WHAT IS THE VALIDITY OF THE INFANT, TODDLER, AND PRESCHOOL SEAM™ INTERVALS, SPECIFICALLY CONTENT AND CONGRUENT VALIDITY?

Correlation of Mean SEAM™ Scores with Age

Two analyses were computed using a subset of the data sample that included children who were known to be typically developing in order to 1) calculate mean SEAM scores across 6-month intervals for all age intervals and 2) calculate correlation of mean SEAM scores with age for the Infant and Toddler Intervals. There was a consistent increase in mean scores across the 6-month age intervals in both the Infant and Toddler Intervals (see Table 7.8). Nonetheless, the Preschool Interval did not demonstrate this increasing trend. Correlations of mean scores with age for the Infant ($r = .354$) and Toddler ($r = .391$) Intervals were moderate and significant at $p < .01$, suggesting that children's scores did increase with age but with some variations, which means children of the same age may have different total scores on the SEAM. Correlation of mean scores with age for the Preschool Interval ($r = .124$) was low and not significant. Lack of significance for children of preschool age might be due to the variability of children's social-emotional skills related to whether they attend preschools or other learning centers and the skills they learn in these settings. Many skills in the social-emotional domain are acquired by infants and toddlers based on developmental maturation rather than experiential learning. SEAM authors also expected that qualitative, rather than quantitative, changes might be observed at the preschool level because children have generally acquired basic social-emotional skills by this age. Age-based differences are observed in the quality and sophistication of their demonstration of these acquired skills.

Table 7.9. Correlations between Social-Emotional Assessment/Evaluation Measure (SEAM™) scores and other related measures

		DECA	ITSEA Compliance	ITSEA Negative Emotion	ITSEA Pro-social	ASQ:SE
Infant SEAM scores	r	.754**	.628**	−.415*	.651**	−.557**
	n	13	27	26	24	860
Toddler SEAM scores	r	NA	.564**	−.261**	.652**	−.516**
	n		119	120	120	162
Preschool SEAM scores	r	NA	NA	NA	NA	−.810**
	n					417

Key: *p < .05; **p < .01; ASQ:SE, Ages & Stages Questionnaires®: Social-Emotional (Squires, Bricker, & Twombly, 2002); DECA, Devereux Early Childhood Assessment Infant-Toddler (Mackrain, LeBuffe, & Powell, 2007); ITSEA, Infant Toddler Social Emotional Assessment (Carter & Briggs-Gowan, 2006).

Concurrent Validity

The Devereux Early Childhood Assessment Infant-Toddler (DECA-IT; Mackrain, LeBuffe, & Powell, 2007), ITSEA (Carter & Briggs-Gowan, 2006), and ASQ:SE (Squires, Bricker, & Twombly, 2002) were used as the criterion measures to examine the concurrent validity of the SEAM. The Infant Interval of the SEAM was compared with the DECA-IT, ITSEA, and ASQ:SE, and the Toddler Interval of the SEAM had ITSEA and ASQ:SE as the criterion measures.

Devereux Early Childhood Assessment Infant-Toddler Correlations for DECA-IT scores with the Infant Interval (*n* = 13) were strong and significant (*r* = .754). Results are shown in Table 7.9.

Infant Toddler Social Emotional Assessment Correlations were strong and significant for both the Infant (*n* = 27) and Toddler (*n* = 120) Intervals for both Compliance and Pro-social domains (see Table 7.9). The number of subjects varied slightly across domains because cases were included only if all items within a domain were scored, thus allowing a total domain score to be calculated. The correlation between Infant Interval scores and the Compliance domain was *r* = .628, and the Toddler Interval was *r* = .564. The correlation with the Pro-social domain was *r* = .651 for the Infant Interval and *r* = .652 for the Toddler Interval. As expected, correlations between the Negative Emotion subscale for both Infant and Toddler Intervals were in a negative direction. Although the Infant Interval results were strong and significant (*r* = −.415), the Toddler Interval results showed a weak correlation (*r* = −.261) with the Negative Emotion subscale.

Ages & Stages Questionnaires®: Social-Emotional Correlations with the ASQ:SE were in a negative direction for both Infant (*n* = 860) and Toddler (*n* = 162) Intervals for the total sample (measuring challenging behaviors in ASQ:SE and competence in SEAM) (see Table 7.9). The correlation between the ASQ:SE and the Infant Interval (*r* = −.557) was strong and significant, and the correlation between the ASQ:SE and the Toddler Interval (*r* = −.516) was moderate/strong and also significant. The correlation between the ASQ:SE and the Preschool (*n* = 417) Interval (*r* = −.810) was also strong and significant. This was the expected outcome because SEAM scores increased with competence and ASQ:SE scores increased as negative behaviors and concerns increased.

QUESTION 4: WHAT IS THE UTILITY OF THE SEAM™ SYSTEM?

The authors collected utility data from 434 caregivers who completed the SEAM. More than 93% of caregivers felt that the SEAM asked appropriate and useful questions. Ninety-one percent of caregivers felt that items were clearly worded. Caregivers indicated they were alerted to new child skills (56% agreed or strongly agreed, whereas 23% had no opinion); 89% indicated that completing the SEAM did not bring up any concerns about their children that they felt they needed to talk to someone about. Caregivers said that it took them an average of 9 minutes to complete the SEAM, indicating a reasonable time for caregiver completion.

Researchers also conducted a written utility survey with 35 practitioners from Part C early intervention programs. Of this group, demographic information was collected from 34 practitioners. Practitioners had an average of 8 years of experience working with children birth through age 5 years. The majority held either a bachelor's (47%) or postgraduate/graduate degree (47%), with 6% holding an associate's degree. Practitioners used a 4-point scale to rate their skill level related to providing mental health services to infants and toddlers and their families, with 1 = *very low* and 4 = *very high*. Four participants (12%) gave themselves a 1 rating; 19 participants (56%) gave a 2 rating; 10 participants (29%) gave a 3 rating; and 1 participant (3%) gave a 4 rating.

Six percent of practitioners used only the Infant Interval of the SEAM; 47% used only the Toddler Interval; and 47% of practitioners used both. Each practitioner completed between 1 and 19 SEAM intervals, with the majority completing 1 to 4. The majority of practitioners (91%) completed the SEAM with families during home visits; whereas others (6%) completed the SEAM in a child care center or in other ways (11%), such as having a caregiver complete it on his or her own at home. Written comments on preferred completion methods revealed a preference for completing the SEAM with caregivers during home visits, through a conversational or interview style that permitted discussion of questions.

Ninety-two percent of practitioners agreed or strongly agreed that SEAM items were clear and easy to understand. Seventy-nine percent ($n = 33$) agreed or strongly agreed that completing the SEAM gave them meaningful information about a child's social-emotional abilities and needs. Sixty percent ($n = 33$) agreed or strongly agreed that they would use the SEAM again; 30% had no opinion; 9% disagreed. Sixty-two percent ($n = 29$) agreed or strongly agreed that they planned to address some of the skills caregivers indicated as intervention goals on the SEAM; 35% had no opinion.

Researchers also conducted two focus groups in order to further understand the utility of the SEAM. The first focus group included 12 teachers and took place in an early child care setting following the interrater reliability study described in which the SEAM was completed by teachers. The second focus group was conducted with five practitioners (home visitors and toddler classroom teachers) from an agency responsible for delivering Part C early intervention services. Participating practitioners in this group completed both the SEAM and the SEAM Family Profile. These practitioners completed between 12 and 41 SEAM protocols each and reported that some caregivers independently completed the SEAM with no problems, while the practitioners administered the SEAM to others in an interview format or in the context of a guided parent group. Focus group questions asked about the benefits and challenges of using the SEAM system with families and included questions such as 1) Did using the SEAM affect your relationship with the families you serve? If so, how? and 2) Did the SEAM give you any new information about the children and families with whom you work?

Although a formal qualitative study was not completed, focus group questions were intended to solicit more in-depth information than the utility surveys provided. The data reported next are summarized from the group conducted with Part C providers who implemented the SEAM in a caregiver-completed format. During this focus group process, facilitators regularly checked for agreement or disagreement among participants. The themes summarized next are those on which participants expressed agreement or which were expressed by the majority of participating practitioners.

Focus group participants preferred the interview format and stressed the importance of having a practitioner involved in SEAM completion in order to clarify items, explain examples, explore concerns, and help caregivers choose appropriate response options. Other themes emerged surrounding the impact of the SEAM on the relationship between practitioners and families. Several practitioners indicated that the SEAM opened up conversations with families that might not otherwise have taken place. One practitioner stated,

"So I think it was a really nice forum for a conversation to learn more about the frequency. Things were more intense than I had realized previously. I hadn't really asked the right questions until I stepped through it."

Practitioners also indicated that they learned new information about families that helped guide future interventions and support children's development. According to one practitioner,

"By doing [the SEAM] with [families], I found some areas that I didn't know were issues for families or where they were having difficult times. So it did help me guide the home visit piece of my service. We never had a conversation about it because the social area wasn't an area that we were too concerned about. It doesn't mean it's an area of delay, but it does mean it's something that's affecting the family that I can help with, which overall helps with overall development."

Finally, practitioners discussed the difficulty of using the SEAM with families whose children had serious concerns of which caregivers were not already aware. They stressed the importance of sensitivity to each family's individual issues and needs and cautioned against having every family independently complete the SEAM, particularly when it might reveal new information that might be emotionally difficult to receive. One practitioner described one such family to whom she had given the SEAM.

"It was a child who we were truly concerned about with autism, and the parent got very emotional because it really brought out the social differences for that family. I hadn't really thought about how much this would affect that particular diagnosis or the ability to see where the discrepancies were. It definitely was a trigger. I would have done it really differently because it really hit them hard, and I felt like it was an emotional effect that I would have liked to have buffered had I really thought about it. And now if I had to do it again, I would do it differently, for sure, or maybe not even do it with that particular family."

FUTURE RESEARCH EFFORTS

The authors have collected objective data in this initial study of the SEAM system to substantiate the SEAM intervals as well as additional utility data gathered through focus groups. The authors used IRT to investigate item functioning and item ordering and conducted classical test analyses in order to perform the validity and reliability studies. Results suggest the SEAM had robust results related to validity, reliability, and utility. Further study is needed, however, with a stratified, randomized national sample to confirm these results. Linked system processes with intervention/curriculum development and program evaluation, including child monitoring and program effectiveness, also need to be studied.

We believe the SEAM is a measure with data that validates its use in the realm of social-emotional assessment and intervention. Research is ongoing; the authors continue to collect and assemble information to examine the validity, reliability, and usefulness of the SEAM. Additional recent research efforts have begun to investigate the SEAM Family Profile as well as the quality of goals written by practitioners using both the SEAM and the SEAM Family Profile. Future research efforts will focus on the effectiveness of the SEAM in monitoring child progress over time.

References

Carter, A.S., & Briggs-Gowan, M.J. (2006). *Infant Toddler Social Emotional Assessment*. San Antonio, TX: Pearson.

Cronbach, L. (1951). Coefficient alpha and the internal structure of tests. *Psychometrika, 16*, 279–334.

Embretson, S., & Reise, S. (2000). *Item response theory for psychologists*. Mahwah, NJ: Lawrence Erlbaum Associates.

Hambleton, R.K., & Swaminathan, H. (1985). *Item response theory: Principles and applications*. Boston, MA: Kluwer-Nijhoff.

Linacre, J.M. (2011). *Winsteps Rasch Measurement Version 3.71* [Software]. Available from http://www.winsteps.com

Mackrain, M., LeBuffe, P., & Powell, G. (2007). *Devereux Early Childhood Assessment for Infants and Toddlers user's guide*. Lewisville, NC: Kaplan Early Learning.

Masters, G.N., & Wright, B.D. (1997). The partial credit model. In W.J. van derLinden & R.K. Hambleton (Eds.), *Handbook of modern item response theory* (pp. 101–122). New York, NY: Springer.

Squires, J., & Bricker, D. (2007). *An activity-based approach to developing young children's social emotional competence*. Baltimore, MD: Paul H. Brookes Publishing Co.

Squires, J., Bricker, D., & Twombly, E. (2002). *The ASQ:SE user's guide*. Baltimore, MD: Paul H. Brookes Publishing Co.

Squires, J., Waddell, M., Clifford, J., Funk, M., Hoselton, R., & Chen, C. (2012a). *Project SEAM: Preventing behavior disorders and improving social-emotional competence for infants and toddlers with disabilities: Final report*. Washington, DC: Institute of Education Sciences.

Squires, J., Waddell, M., Clifford, J., Funk, M., Hoselton, R., & Chen, C. (2012b). Psychometric study of the Infant and Toddler Intervals of the Social Emotional Assessment Measure. *Topics in Early Childhood Special Education*. doi:10.1177/0271121412463445

Appendix A
SEAM™ Benchmarks and Items

Age interval		Benchmark		Item
Infant	C-1.0	Baby participates in healthy interactions.	1.1	Baby shows interest in you and other familiar caregivers.
			1.2	Baby lets you know if she needs help or comfort.
			1.3	Baby responds to you and other familiar caregivers.
			1.4	Baby initiates and responds to communications.
	C-2.0	Baby expresses a range of emotions.	2.1	Baby smiles at you.
			2.2	Baby smiles at familiar people.
			2.3	Baby smiles and laughs at sights and sounds.
	C-3.0	Baby regulates own social-emotional responses with caregiver support.	3.1	Baby calms down after exciting activity.
			3.2	Baby responds to your soothing when upset.
			3.3	Baby soothes self when distressed.
	C-4.0	Baby begins to show empathy for others.	4.1	Baby mimics your facial expressions.
			4.2	Baby looks at and notices you and other familiar caregivers.
			4.3	Baby looks at and notices others' emotional responses.
			4.4	Baby responds to another's distress, seeking comfort for self.
	C-5.0	Baby attends to and engages with others.	5.1	Baby looks at or toward sounds and visual events.
			5.2	Baby makes eye contact with you and others.
			5.3	Baby focuses on events shown by you and others.
			5.4	Baby shares attention and events with you.

Age interval	Benchmark		Item	
	C-6.0	Baby explores hands and feet and surroundings.	6.1 6.2 6.3 6.4	Baby explores hands and feet. Baby explores toys and materials. Baby explores surroundings. Baby crawls or walks a short distance away from you.
	C-7.0	Baby displays a positive self-image.	7.1 7.2 7.3	Baby calls attention to self. Baby laughs or smiles at own image or picture of self. Baby recognizes own name.
	C-8.0	Baby regulates activity level.	8.1 8.2 8.3	Baby participates in simple routines and games with you. Baby engages in motor activities for several minutes or longer. Baby looks at books or pictures for several minutes or longer.
	C-9.0	Baby cooperates with daily routines and requests.	9.1 9.2 9.3	Baby opens mouth for food. Baby follows simple routines with your help. Baby cooperates with diaper and clothing changes.
	C-10.0	Baby shows a range of adaptive skills.	10.1 10.2 10.3 10.4	Baby eliminates (pees and poops) on a regular schedule. Baby eats and gains weight on schedule. Baby sleeps with few problems. Baby eats a variety of age-appropriate foods.
Toddler	C-1.0	Toddler participates in healthy interactions.	1.1 1.2 1.3 1.4	Toddler lets you know if he needs help, attention, or comfort. Toddler initiates and responds to affection. Toddler talks and plays with people whom he knows well. Toddler initiates and responds when you communicate with her.
	C-2.0	Toddler expresses a range of emotions.	2.1 2.2 2.3 2.4	Toddler smiles and laughs. Toddler expresses a range of emotions in a variety of ways. Toddler identifies own emotions, with your help. Toddler identifies own emotions.
	C-3.0	Toddler regulates own social-emotional responses.	3.1 3.2 3.3	Toddler responds to soothing when upset. Toddler can settle self down after periods of exciting activity. Toddler can calm self when upset.

Age interval	Benchmark		Item	
	C-4.0	Toddler begins to show empathy for others.	4.1	Toddler matches response to others' emotional responses.
			4.2	Toddler tries to comfort others when they are upset.
			4.3	Toddler uses words to talk about another child's emotions.
	C-5.0	Toddler shares attention and engages with others.	5.1	Toddler makes eye contact with caregivers and peers.
			5.2	Toddler focuses on events that you show him.
			5.3	Toddler greets you and other familiar people.
			5.4	Toddler shares in daily activities.
			5.5	Toddler plays alongside other children.
	C-6.0	Toddler demonstrates independence.	6.1	Toddler tries new tasks before seeking help.
			6.2	Toddler can separate from you in familiar environment with minimal distress.
			6.3	Toddler explores new environments while maintaining some contact.
	C-7.0	Toddler displays a positive self-image.	7.1	Toddler points to self in picture.
			7.2	Toddler tells you what she did or accomplished.
			7.3	Toddler knows personal information.
	C-8.0	Toddler regulates own attention and activity level.	8.1	Toddler moves from one activity to another without problems.
			8.2	Toddler participates in simple games.
			8.3	Toddler stays with motor activities for 5 minutes or longer.
			8.4	Toddler looks at book or listens to story for 5 minutes or longer.
	C-9.0	Toddler cooperates with daily routines and requests.	9.1	Toddler cooperates with simple requests.
			9.2	Toddler follows routines.
	C-10.0	Toddler shows a range of adaptive skills.	10.1	Toddler eats and feeds self a variety of foods without problems.
			10.2	Toddler accepts changes in routines and settings.
			10.3	Toddler falls and remains asleep with few problems.
			10.4	Toddler shows an interest in using the toilet.

Age interval	Benchmark		Item	
Preschool	C-1.0	Preschool-age child demonstrates healthy interactions with others.	1.1	Child shows affection toward you and other familiar adults and children.
			1.2	Child talks and plays with you and other familiar adults and children.
			1.3	Child uses words to let you know if he needs help, attention, or comfort.
			1.4	Child plays with other children.
			1.5	Child shares and takes turns with other children.
	C-2.0	Preschool-age child expresses a range of emotions.	2.1	Child smiles and laughs.
			2.2	Child expresses a range of emotions using a variety of strategies.
			2.3	Child describes emotions of others.
			2.4	Child identifies own emotions.
	C-3.0	Preschool-age child regulates social-emotional responses.	3.1	Child can calm self after periods of exciting activity.
			3.2	Child responds to peer's or caregiver's soothing when upset.
			3.3	Child can calm self when upset within 5 minutes.
			3.4	Child remains calm in disappointing situations.
	C-4.0	Preschool-age child shows empathy for others.	4.1	Child responds appropriately to others' emotional responses.
			4.2	Child tries to comfort others when they are upset.
	C-5.0	Preschool-age child shares and engages with others.	5.1	Child focuses on or joins activities.
			5.2	Child greets adults and peers.
			5.3	Child cooperates in play or when completing a task.
			5.4	Child participates appropriately in group activities.
	C-6.0	Preschool-age child demonstrates independence.	6.1	Child explores new materials and settings.
			6.2	Child can leave you without distress.
			6.3	Child tries new task before seeking help.
			6.4	Child stays with or returns to challenging activities.
	C-7.0	Preschool-age child displays a positive self-image.	7.1	Child shows off work and takes pride in accomplishments.
			7.2	Child makes positive statements about self.
			7.3	Child knows personal information.

Age interval	Benchmark		Item	
	C-8.0	Preschool-age child regulates attention and activity level.	8.1	Child regulates activity level to match setting.
			8.2	Child participates in early literacy activities.
			8.3	Child stays with motor activity for 10 minutes or longer.
			8.4	Child moves from one activity to another without problems.
			8.5	Child participates in games with others.
	C-9.0	Preschool-age child cooperates with daily routines and requests.	9.1	Child follows routines and rules.
			9.2	Child does what he is asked to do.
			9.3	Child responds appropriately when corrected by adults.
	C-10.0	Preschool-age child shows a range of adaptive skills.	10.1	Child solves problems to meet needs.
			10.2	Child manages changes in settings and conditions.
			10.3	Child keeps self safe in potentially dangerous conditions.
			10.4	Child feeds self and eats a variety of foods without a problem.
			10.5	Child dresses self.
			10.6	Child uses the toilet appropriately.
			10.7	Child goes to bed and falls asleep without a problem.

Appendix B
SEAM™ Family Profile Benchmarks and Items

Age interval		Benchmark		Item
Infant	F-1.0	Responding to my baby's needs	1.1	I understand my baby's nonverbal communication and know how to respond.
			1.2	I understand my baby's verbal communication and know how to respond.
			1.3	I know how to help my baby calm down.
	F-2.0	Providing activities and playing with my baby	2.1	I provide books, toys, and playthings that are safe and that my baby enjoys.
			2.2	I know games and activities that my baby enjoys.
	F-3.0	Providing predictable schedule/routines and appropriate environment for my baby	3.1	I create and follow routines that make eating enjoyable and satisfying for me and my baby.
			3.2	I provide a nap and sleeping schedule/ routine for my baby that is predictable and appropriate for her age.
			3.3	I use daily activities as playtime or make time each day to play with my baby.
	F-4.0	Providing my baby with a safe home and play environment	4.1	I have done a safety check on my home to make it safe for my baby.
			4.2	I have a safe way to transport my baby.
			4.3	I know ways to keep my baby safe throughout the day.
			4.4	I have someone I trust who can help take care of my baby.
			4.5	I have access to health care for my baby.
			4.6	I know how to manage feelings of anger or frustration that may occur while I am with my baby.

Age interval	Benchmark		Item	
Toddler	F-1.0	Responding to my child's needs	1.1	I understand my child's nonverbal communication and know how to respond.
			1.2	I understand my child's verbal communication and know how to respond.
			1.3	I know how to support my child's emotional needs.
			1.4	I use positive comments and language with my child.
			1.5	I know how to successfully redirect my child's inappropriate behaviors.
			1.6	I understand why my child engages in inappropriate behaviors and know how to modify the environment.
	F-2.0	Providing activities that match my child's developmental level	2.1	I provide my child books, toys, and playthings that match her developmental level.
			2.2	I know the age-appropriate games that my child enjoys.
	F-3.0	Providing predictable schedule/routines and appropriate environment for my child	3.1	I provide a mealtime routine for my child that is predictable and appropriate for her age.
			3.2	I provide a rest and sleeping routine for my child that is predictable and appropriate for his age.
			3.3	I provide my child with predictable limits and consequences.
			3.4	I take time each day to play with my child.
	F-4.0	Providing a safe home and play environment for my child	4.1	I have done a safety check on my home to make it safe for my child.
			4.2	I have a safe way to transport my child.
			4.3	I am able to provide my child with safe care and supervision.
			4.4	I have access to regular medical and dental care for my child.
			4.5	I know how to manage my own feelings of anger and frustration that come up while with my child.
Preschool	F-1.0	Responding to my child's needs	1.1	I understand my child's nonverbal communication and know how to respond.
			1.2	I understand my child's verbal communication and know how to respond.
			1.3	I know how to support my child's emotional needs.
			1.4	I use positive comments and language with my child.
			1.5	I know how to successfully redirect my child's inappropriate behaviors.
			1.6	I understand why my child engages in inappropriate behaviors and know how to modify the environment.

Age interval	Benchmark		Item	
	F-2.0	Providing activities that match my child's developmental level	2.1	I provide my child with books, toys, and activities that match his developmental level.
			2.2	I know the age-appropriate games that my child enjoys.
	F-3.0	Providing predictable schedule/routines and appropriate environment for my child	3.1	I provide a mealtime routine for my child that is predictable and appropriate for his age.
			3.2	I provide a rest and sleeping routine for my child that is predictable and appropriate for her age.
			3.3	I provide my child with predictable limits and consequences.
			3.4	I take time each day to play with my child.
	F-4.0	Providing a safe home and play environment for my child	4.1	I have done a safety check on my home to make it safe for my child.
			4.2	I have a safe way to transport my child.
			4.3	I am able to provide my child with safe care and supervision.
			4.4	I have access to regular medical and dental care for my child.
			4.5	I know how to manage my own feelings of anger and frustration that come up when I am with my child.

Index

Tables and figures are indicated by *t* or *f*, respectively.